English for Medicine and Health Sciences

English for Medicine and Health Sciences

Shehdeh Fareh, PhD
Professor in Linguistics and TEFL
Director of the English Language Center
Department of English Language and Literature
Author of a series of books for TEFL
University of Sharjah

Inaam A.F. Hamadi, MA
Applied Linguistics
Certificate of Competency in Teaching and Learning from the
Institute of Academic Leadership
Department of English Language and Literature
University of Sharjah

ELSEVIER

ELSEVIER

Elsevier Limited

7th Circle, Zahran Plaza, 7th Floor, PO Box 140825, Amman, 11814, Jordan

English for Medicine and Health Sciences, by Shehdeh Fareh and Inaam A.F. Hamadi

Copyright © 2017 Elsevier Limited.

ISBN: 978-0-7020-7550-6
e-ISBN: 978-0-7020-7551-3

Notices

Practitioners and researchers must always rely on their own experience and knowledge in evaluating and using any information, methods, compounds or experiments described herein. Because of rapid advances in the medical sciences, in particular, independent verification of diagnoses and drug dosages should be made. To the fullest extent of the law, no responsibility is assumed by Elsevier, authors, editors or contributors for any injury and/or damage to persons or property as a matter of products liability, negligence or otherwise, or from any use or operation of any methods, products, instructions, or ideas contained in the material herein.

Content Strategist: Rasheed Roussan
Sr Project Manager—Education Solutions: Shabina Nasim
Content Development Specialist: Amani Bazzari
Project Manager: Nayagi Athmanathan
Cover Designer: Milind Majgaonkar

Printed in India

Dedication

This book is gratefully dedicated to:
Our sincere wives and children for their patience
and encouragement,
our wonderful readers and colleagues,
all those who helped us produce this book.

Reviewers

Hussam Rajab, PhD
Professor
Head of Research Unit
English Language Institute (ELI)
King Abdulaziz University (KAU)
Jeddah, Saudi Arabia

Ghada A. Abdel-Hamid, MD
Associate professor of anatomy
Faculty of Medicine
Suez Canal University
Egypt

Sesin Kocagoz, PhD
Professor
Acıbadem University School of Medicine
Head of Department of Infectious Diseases and Clinical Microbiology
Co-Coordinator of Medical English
Istanbul, Turkey

Foreword

There is an urgent need for a comprehensive book such as *English for Medicine and Health Sciences*. This book is one of the few to address the specific needs of non-native speakers who are attending medical education institutes.

One of the book's landmark features is its ability to communicate complex structures of medical English in a clear and engaging manner, with the learner at the core of the pedagogical context of the book.

With an array of key terminologies, medical roots, and illustrative examples, the book is an essential reference that brings together medical knowledge and language skills indispensable to medicine and health sciences students today.

Offering relevant and cutting-edge literature pertaining to medical English, including an English–English–Arabic Glossary, the book is a hands-on tool for leveraging the students' understanding of the basic principles of written and spoken English required to start a career in medicine and health care.

Moreover, the book is equally invaluable to medical English instructors who are keen to provide the most relevant linguistic material to their students.

I believe that this book offers an opportunity for the students to develop a comprehensive and up-to-date understanding of medical English, offered by a team of highly experienced medical English instructors.

PROF QUTAYBA HAMID, MD, PhD, FRCP, FRS
Dean, College of Medicine
University of Sharjah

Preface

English for Medical and Health Sciences

In order to be successful professionals, students in the fields of medicine and health sciences need to be competent in using medical terminology. They need to familiarize themselves with as many medical terms as possible in order to function properly in their study and future careers. This means that students should know the meanings of medical terms used in their fields and how they are composed. Furthermore, they need to enhance their essential language skills including reading, writing and speaking. *English for Medical and Health Sciences* is especially designed to meet these basic needs. It consists of five chapters that cover the structure of medical terms, prefixes, suffixes, body structure, and body systems. Each chapter consists of at least 10 basic components as follows:

- Medical terms: Lists of terms relevant to the content of each chapter are provided and their meanings are also given. Prefixes and suffixes are also explained in detail with illustrative examples.
- Practice exercises: Activities are provided after each section to check the students' understanding. Teachers can use these activities as formative assessment tools.
- Focus on vocabulary: This part of each chapter provides students with two lists of academic vocabulary that are essential for developing students' lexical competence. Furthermore, this part provides students with 20 medical collocations with illustrative examples and practice activities. Students are also introduced to medical idioms commonly used in their fields.
- Focus on reading: This section aims at promoting students' abilities to handle and comprehend medical texts. It also familiarizes them with medical terms used in context.
- Focus on grammar: Each chapter handles a certain grammatical notion that is common in medical and scientific texts.
- Focus on speaking: This part aims at enhancing the students' oral communication skills. Students are trained to speak in clinical contexts with each other, with their instructors, and with patients.

- Focus on writing: Writing is a complex skill that needs to be developed through a systematic training. Students are given practice in writing definitions of terms and in writing referral letters throughout the five chapters of the book.
- Pronunciation list: New medical terms in each chapter are listed at the end of the respective chapters for students to pronounce. They are also encouraged to know their meanings. Students can listen to the proper pronunciation from their instructors or from a CD especially prepared for this purpose.
- Review exercises: These exercises provide students with more practice activities on all the components of the chapter. Teachers can also use them as summative assessment tools.
- Case studies: Each chapter provides one or two case studies for students to learn from. Case studies present clinical descriptions and diagnoses of certain medical cases.
- Glossary of medical terms and their meanings in English and Arabic for Arab students.
- Teacher's manual: This guidebook offers teachers with answers to the practice activities and review exercises in each chapter. It also contains quizzes and tests that the teacher can use. Finally, it contains a number of reading comprehension texts that can be used in tests and quizzes, and for training as well.

The distinctive features of *English for Medical and Health Sciences* can be summed up as follows:

- Provides exhaustive lists of medical roots, combining forms, prefixes, and suffixes with illustrative examples.
- Offers an integrated course that combines medical knowledge with essential language skills.
- Focuses on developing students' reading skills in medical contexts.
- Develops students' oral communications skills necessary for interaction in their fields.
- Reinforces students' academic vocabulary needed for effective communication.
- Promotes students' awareness and competence of medical collocations and idioms.
- Enhances students' writing skills in their medical fields.
- Develops students' grammatical competence in areas relevant to their medical majors.
- Provides ample and frequent practice and review exercises in each chapter.

- Provides teachers with sample quizzes, tests, and answer keys for each chapter.
- Provides a glossary of the major medical terms.

The outstanding features of this well-organized book help students develop their medical knowledge and linguistic competence as well. These integrated skills can hardly be found in any existing textbook in this field.

Acknowledgments

First and foremost, all thanks and praise goes to Allah, who granted us the knowledge and power to write this book.

We wish to express our thanks and gratitude to all those who helped us in producing the first edition of *English for Medical and Health Sciences*.

Thanks to the development team and Amani Bazzari who were keen to produce the book in its best shape.

Thanks are also due to the book reviewers for their valuable feedback that improved the quality of the book.

Special thanks and appreciation are due to our students in the medical colleges who volunteered to read the chapters of the book and give us their feedback that was highly appreciated since it reflected the students' views regarding the contents of the book.

Dr Mustafa Hammadeh, from Twam Hospital, was our consultant in all medical issues. His assistance was invaluable.

We would also like to thank Mr Rasheed Roussan and his team for their follow-up and encouragement.

Table of Contents

CHAPTER 1

Medical Terminology

LEARNING OUTCOMES

At the end of this chapter, students are expected to be able to:
1. explain the need for medical terms
2. define the constituents of medical terms: root, suffix, and prefix
3. define medical combining forms
4. analyze medical terms into their constituents
5. construct medical terms by applying general rules
6. use certain medical collocations and academic words properly
7. pronounce medical terms properly
8. skim and scan medical texts for main ideas and details
9. paraphrase a sentence or a paragraph
10. prepare an oral presentation

LANGUAGE OF MEDICINE

Terminology is the set of terms, expressions, or symbols associated with a certain discipline of study, profession, or activity. Developing a functional competence in terminology is an essential component of being able to work in a given field or profession. Medical terminology is the variety of language that health care professionals and providers use in practicing their careers. Medical terms constitute a standardized means of communication among health care providers because all such specialists use special terminology to describe human body, diseases, symptoms, diagnostic procedures, drug administration, and treatment in the fields of medicine, nursing, pharmacy, dentistry, physiotherapy, medical lab sciences, clinical nutrition, and dietetics, environmental health sciences, and medical diagnostic imaging. Medical terms are used in both speaking and writing during the process of communication between health care professionals and their clients. Therefore, it is essential for students in any medical profession to learn the meanings of medical terms pertaining to each one's career. It is also necessary to learn how to pronounce and spell medical terms properly because mistakes in such fields are intolerable. The significance of learning medical terms stems from the following reasons:

- Medical terms enable health care workers to communicate efficiently with each other and with their patients in one language.
- They ensure complete and mutual understanding of patients' issues, including diagnosis and treatment procedures.
- Medical terms help us decipher complex information because they are made up of roots, prefixes, and suffixes that generally have fixed meanings to all workers in health care careers.
- Medical terms facilitate the process of documentation and make it easy and fast due to the frequent use of abbreviations in recording medical information.

It has become clear that possessing an adequate functional knowledge of medical terms is indispensable to all people working in health-related disciplines. Knowledge of medical terms involves a number of aspects such as knowing the meaning/s of a medical term, its structure, its derived forms, spelling, and pronunciation.

Medical terms are almost universal because most of them are derived from Latin or Greek origins. Table 1.1 provides samples of modern medical terms and their

Table 1.1 Latin and Greek Origins of Some Current Medical Terms

Current Term	Origin
artery	Latin *arteria*; Greek *arteria*
cardi(o) the heart	Greek *kardia*
cell	Latin *cella*
ligament	Latin *ligamentum*
nephropathia	Greek *nephros*
ventricle	Latin *venter*
umbilicus	Latin *umbilic*
tendon	Latin *tendo*
sinus	Latin *sinus*
vein	Latin *vena*
nerve	Latin *nervus*
hernia	Latin *hernia*
gastr	Greek *gaster* (stomach)
ovary	Greek *oophor*
cancer	Greek carcin

Latin or Greek origins. Learning medical vocabulary is a strenuous and highly demanding process because it is always changing and developing. Although most medical terms are based on classical Latin and Greek roots, they are no longer restricted to such origins. Many medical terms nowadays have been borrowed from ordinary English words such as *scanning*, *screening*, and *bypass operation*. In order to learn the meanings of medical terms, students need to familiarize themselves with the way medical terms are structured and created. A medical term is usually composed of a root that carries the basic sense of the term to which prefixes and suffixes may be added.

MEDICAL TERMS

Constituents of Medical Terms: Roots, Suffixes, Prefixes, and Combining Forms

Roots

The primary constituent of each medical term is the root that carries its basic meaning. Prefixes and suffixes can be added to the root to modify its meaning.

A root is the part of a word that carries its basic meaning. The root in medical terms cannot stand alone to give a complete meaning. A prefix or a suffix may be added to it in order to make a full term that has meaning. This is due to

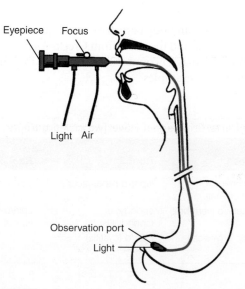

FIGURE 1.1 Gastroscopy: visual examination of the stomach.

the fact that most medical roots are borrowed from different source languages such as Latin and Greek. In the word *gastroscopy,* for example, the root is *gastr* (stomach) and *-scopy is a suffix* (visual examination). Adding the meaning of the suffix to that of the root will make up the entire meaning of the medical term *gastroscopy* (visual examination of the stomach).

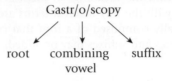

A medical term may consist of one or more roots but only one suffix, as shown in Table 1.2. We can only add a prefix whenever we need to modify the meaning of the root.

Table 1.2 Medical Terms with One or More Roots	
One root	**hem**/o/globin
Two roots	**electr**/o/**cardi**/o/gram
Three roots	**ot**/o/**rhin**/o/**laryng**/o/logy
Four roots	**esophag**/o/**gastr**/o/**duoden**/o/**jejun**/o/stomy

It is worth noting that certain body parts have more than one word root, because one root comes from Latin and the other from Greek. You should be familiar with both roots because you may encounter both of them in your study. Table 1.3 provides some illustrative examples.

Body Part/Organ	Root 1	Root 2	Root 3	Root 4
abdomen	abdomin/o (abdominal)	lapar/o (laparoscopy)	celi/o (celiac)	
backbone	vertebr/o (vertebral)	spondyl/o (spondylitis)	spin/o (spinal column)	
urinary bladder	vesic/o (vesical)	cyst/o (cystitis)		

Table 1.3 Body Parts/Organs that Have Two or More Roots

Table 1.3 Body Parts/Organs that Have Two or More Roots—cont'd

Body Part/ Organ	Root 1	Root 2	Root 3	Root 4
blood vessel	angi/o (angiogram)	vas/o (vasoconstriction)	vascul/o (vascular)	
breast	mamm/o (mammogram)	mast/o (mastectomy)		
eardrum	tympan/o (tympanic)	myring/o (myringotomy)		
eye	ocul/o (ocular)	ophthalm/o (ophthalmoscope)	opt/o (optician)	optic/o (optical)
heart	coron/o (coronary)	cardi/o (cardiology)		
kidney	ren/o (renal)	nephr/o (nephritis)		
lung	pulmon/o (pulmonary)	pneumon/o (pneumonectomy)	pulm/o (pulmoaortic)	
mouth	or/o (oral)	stomat/o (stomatitis)		
muscle	muscul/o (muscular)	my/o (myoma)	myos/o (myositis)	
nose	nas/o (nasal)	rhin/o (rhinitis)		
ovary	ovari/o (ovarian)	oophor/o (oophorectomy)		
skin	cutane/o (cutaneous)	dermat/o (dermatitis)	derm/o (dermal)	epitheli/o (epithelial)
uterus	uter/o (uterine)	hyster/o (hysterectomy)	metri/o (endometrium)	
vagina	vagin/o (vaginal)	colp/o (colposcopy)		
vein	ven/o (venous)	phleb/o (phlebitis)		
testes	orch/o (orchiectomy)	orchid/o (orchidoplasty)	orchi/o (orchiopexy)	
blood	hem/o (hemoglobin)	hemat/o (hematorrhagia)		
colon	col/o (colostomy)	colon/o (colonoscopy)		
pituitary gland	pituitary/o (hypopituitarism)	hypophys/o (hypophysis)		

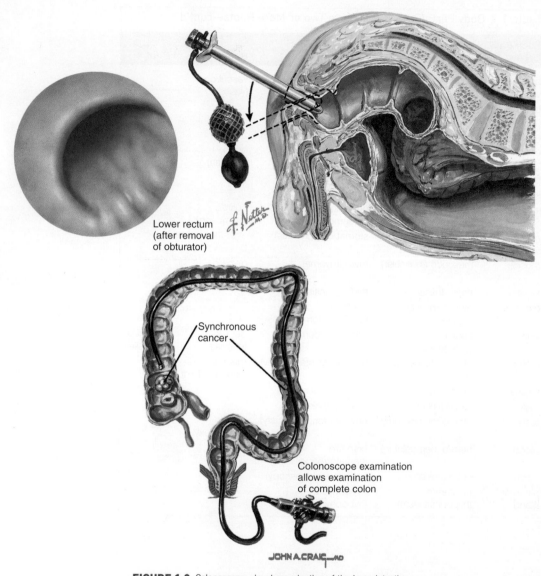

Lower rectum
(after removal
of obturator)

Synchronous
cancer

Colonoscope examination
allows examination
of complete colon

FIGURE 1.2 Colonoscopy: visual examination of the large intestine.

Common Combining Forms

Combining Form	Meaning	Medical Term	Meaning
angi/o	blood vessel	angiogram	_____
arthr/o	joint	arthritis	_____
bronch/o	bronchial tube	bronchoscopy	_____
carcin/o	cancer	carcinoma	_____
cardi/o	heart	cardiologist	_____
chron/o	time	chronic	_____
cephal/o	brain	cephalic	_____
cerebr/o	largest part of the brain	cerebrosclerosis	_____
cervic/o	neck	cervical	_____
col/o	large intestine	colostomy	_____
cyst/o	urinary bladder	cystitis	_____
cyt/o	cell	cytologist	_____
derm/o	skin	transdermal	_____
dermat/o	skin	dermatologist	_____
duoden/o	the first part of the small intestine	duodenoscope	_____
electr/o	electricity	electrocardiogram	_____
encephal/o	brain	encephalitis	_____
enter/o	intestine	gastroenterology	_____
erythr/o	red	erythrocytosis	_____
esophag/o	food tube	esophagoscopy	_____
gastr/o	stomach	gastric	_____
gingiv/o	gum	gingivitis	_____
glyc/o	sugar	hyperglycemia	_____
gnos/o	knowledge	prognosis	_____
		diagnosis	_____
gynec/o	woman	gynecologist	_____
hem/o hemat/o	blood	hemoglobin	_____
		hematoma	_____
hepat/o	liver	hepatoma	_____
hyster/o	uterus	hysterectomy	_____
lapar/o	abdomen	laparoscope	_____
laryng/o	larynx (voice box)	laryngectomy	_____
leuk/o	white	leukemia	_____
		leukocytosis	_____
mamm/o	breast	mammogram	_____
mast/o	breast	mastectomy	_____

Combining Form	Meaning	Medical Term	Meaning
metri/o	uterus	endometrium	_____
my/o	muscle	myoma	_____
nephr/o	kidney	nephrologist	_____
neur/o	nerve	neuralgia	_____
onc/o	tumor	oncologist	_____
oophor/o	ovary	oophorectomy	_____
ophthalm/o	eye	ophthalmologist	_____
oste/o	bone	osteomyelitis	_____
ot/o	ear	otorhinolaryngology	_____
ovari/o	ovary	ovariopathy	_____
path/o	disease	pathologist	_____
phleb/o	vein	phlebotomy	_____
pneumon/o	lung	pneumonia	_____
psych/o	mind	psychology	_____
pulm/o	lung	pulmonary	_____
radi/o	radiation	radiology	_____
ren/o	kidney	renal	_____
rhin/o	nose	rhinorrhea	_____
sacr/o	lower back	sacral	_____
sarc/o	flesh	myosarcoma	_____
spin/o	vertebral column	spinal	_____
trache/o	windpipe	tracheostomy	_____
throrac/o	chest	thoracotomy	_____
thromb/o	clotting	thrombosis	_____
ur/o	urine or urea	uremia	_____
vascul/o	blood vessel	vascular	_____

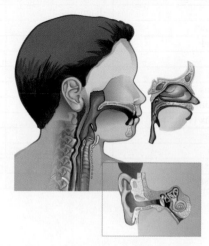

FIGURE 1.3 Otorhinolaryngology: study of ear, nose, and larynx.

Suffixes

A **suffix** is a letter or group of letters added to the end of a word to change its meaning or to produce a new word (part of speech). For example, if the suffix *-tomy* (cutting into) is added to the root *gastr*, the resulting term *gastrotomy* will mean incision into the stomach. However, if the suffix *-ectomy* is added to the same root, the resulting term *gastrectomy* will mean excision of the stomach. Moreover, adding *-al* to the root *dent* (noun) produces *dental* (adjective).

Notice the difference between *neuralgia, neuritis,* and *neuroplasty*. The meaning of each term differs from that of the other because of the different suffixes added to the same root *neur* which means nerve. The suffix *-algia* means having pain; *-itis* means inflammation; and finally *-plasty* means plastic repair. The first word means condition of having pain in the nerve; the second means inflammation of the nerve and third means plastic repair of the nerve. Table 1.4 provides examples of commonly used but confused suffixes.

Table 1.4 Commonly Used but Confused Suffixes

Suffix	Meaning	Example	Meaning
-tome	instrument to incise (cutting into)	microtome	instrument for cutting thin sections of tissues for microscopic study
-tomy	incision (the process of cutting into)	laparotomy	incision into the abdomen
-ectomy	excision (the process of removal)	adenectomy	excision of a gland
-stomy	opening to the outside of the body (with one root)	tracheostomy	opening of the windpipe to the outside of the body
-stomy	communication (with more than one root)	colocolostomy	communication between two unconnected parts of the large intestine (anastomosis)
-scope	instrument to visually examine	arthroscope	instrument to visually examine joints
-scopy	visual examination	ophthalmoscopy	visual examination of eyes
-logy	study of	gynecology	study of women's diseases
-logist	specialist in the study and treatment of	nephrologist	specialist in the study of kidneys

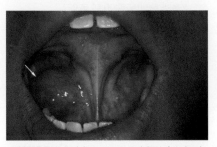

FIGURE 1.4 Adenectomy excision of a gland.

It is worth noting that medical terms are briefly defined throughout the entire book.

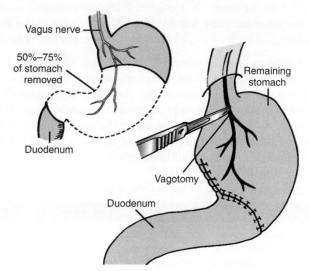

FIGURE 1.5 Gastroduodenostomy: communication between the stomach and first part of the small intestine.

Table 1.5 Terms Using the Suffix -*Scopy* (Visual Examination of)	
Medical Term	**Meaning**
bronchoscopy	visual examination of the bronchial tubes
laryngoscopy	visual examination of the larynx
laparoscopy	visual examination of the abdomen
gastroscopy	visual examination of the stomach
arthroscopy	visual examination of joints
cystoscopy	visual examination of the urinary bladder
ophthalmoscopy	visual examination of eyes
otoscopy	visual examination of ears
sigmoidoscopy	visual examination of the sigmoid colon
rhinoscopy	visual examination of the nose
uroscopy	visual examination of the urinary tract
colonoscopy	visual examination of the large intestine
esophagoscopy	visual examination of the esophagus

Table 1.6 Terms Using the Suffix -*Logist*

Medical Term	Meaning
cardiologist	specialist in the study and treatment of the heart diseases
dermatologist	specialist in the study of skin
oncologist	specialist in the study of tumors
nephrologist	specialist in the study of the kidneys
gynecologist	specialist in the study of women's diseases
trichologist	specialist in the study of hair
urologist	specialist in the study of the urinary system
hematologist	specialist in the study of the blood
biologist	specialist in the study of living tissues
otorhinolaryngologist	specialist in the study of the ear, nose, and larynx
ophthalmologist	specialist in the study of eyes
endocrinologist	specialist in the study of the endocrine system
gastroenterologist	specialist in the study of the stomach and intestine

Commonly Used Suffixes

Suffixes	Meaning	Medical term	Meaning
-al	pertaining to	renal	_____
-ac	pertaining to	cardiac	_____
-algia	pain	otalgia	_____
-algesia	pain	analgesia	_____
-cyte	cell	erythrocyte	_____
-emia	blood condition	uremia	_____
-globin	protein	hemoglobin	_____
-gram	record of	mammogram	_____
-ia	condition of	myalgia	_____
-ic	pertaining to	metric	_____
-ics	medical specialty	orthopedics	_____
-ist	medical specialist	anesthetist	_____
-ism	state of	hypothyroidism	_____
-itis	inflammation	encephalitis	_____
-megaly	enlargement	hepatomegaly	_____
-oma	tumor/mass	hepatoma	_____
		hematoma	_____
		nephroma	_____
-opsy	viewing	autopsy	_____
-osis	abnormal condition of	stenosis	_____
		sclerosis	_____
-pathy	disease	cardiomyopathy	_____
-sis	state of	diagnosis	_____

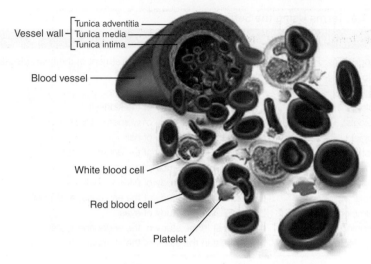

Tunica adventitia
Vessel wall — Tunica media
Tunica intima

Blood vessel

White blood cell

Red blood cell

Platelet

FIGURE 1.6 Erythrocyte: red blood cells.

It is worth noting that sometimes there might be two or more suffixes that have the same meaning but they are not interchangeable. That is to say, where one is used, the other cannot. For example, the suffixes *-opsia* and *-opia* mean vision, but we can only say *diplopia* (double vision) not *diplopsia*.

Prefixes

A **prefix** is a letter or a group of letters attached to the beginning of a root to modify its meaning. For example, the term *hyperglycemia* consists of a prefix (hyper), a root (glyc), and a suffix (-emia).

Consider the following examples and note the different meaning that results when a new prefix is added to the same root.

Prefix	Medical Term	Meaning
hemi-	hemiplegia	paralysis of one side of the body
para-	paraplegia	condition of having lower half paralysis
quadri-	quadriplegia	condition of having paralysis in the four limbs
pan-	panplegia	condition of having total paralysis
pseudo-	pseudoplegia	condition of having false paralysis

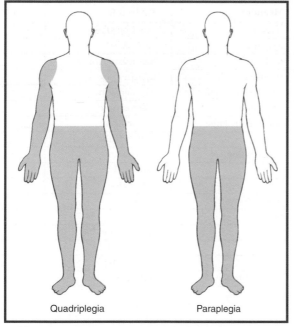

Quadriplegia   Paraplegia

FIGURE 1.7 Quadriplegia: paralysis of the four limbs of the body.

The root **cardi** may be preceded by two different prefixes. The addition of *brady-* (slow) and *tachy-* (rapid) to the same root results in two different terms: **brady/ card/ia** (having slow heart rate) and **tachy/card/ia** (rapid heart rate). Similarly, the root *later* can be preceded by the prefixes *bi-* and *uni-* as in **bi/later/al**, which means pertaining to both sides, and **uni/later/al**, which means pertaining to one side.

Commonly Used Prefixes

Prefix	Meaning	Medical term	Meaning
a-/an-	not	apnea	_____
		anemia	_____
ante-	before	antenatal	_____
anti-	against	antibiotic	_____
ab-	away from	abnormal	_____
ad-	toward	adduct	_____
auto-	self	autopsy	_____
brady-	slow	bradycardia	_____
dia-	through/complete	diameter	_____
		diarrhea	_____
dys-	painful/difficult	dyspnea	_____
	poor/abnormal	dysuria	_____
endo-	within	endocrine glands	_____

Prefix	Meaning	Medical term	Meaning
exo-	outside	exocrine glands	_____
eu-	easy/true	eupnea	_____
hemi-	half	hemigastrectomy	_____
hyper-	excessive	hypertension	_____
hypo-	less than normal	hypotension	_____
macro-	very large	macroscopic	_____
mega-	abnormally large	megacolon	_____
multi-	many	multicellular	_____
peri-	surrounding	periosteum	_____
post-	after	postnatal	_____
pre-	before	prenatal	_____
pro-	before/forward	prodrome	_____
re-	back	resection	_____
retro-	behind	retrouterine	_____
sub-	below	sublingual	_____
tachy-	rapid	tachycardia	_____
trans-	across/through	transfusion	_____

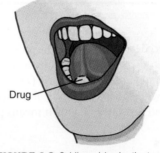

Drug

FIGURE 1.8 Sublingual (under the tongue).

When a suffix starting with a consonant is added to a root ending with a consonant, a vowel is added between the root and the suffix in order to ease the articulation of the resulting form. This vowel is referred to as the **combining vowel**. The root plus the combining vowel are called the **combining form**. The term *cystoscope*, for example, consists of the root *cyst-*, a combining vowel -*o*- and the suffix -*scope*. However, the combining vowel is omitted if the suffix starts with a vowel as in *gastrectomy* (gastr + ectomy), *cephalic* (cephal + ic), *adenitis* (aden + itis), *neuralgia* (neur + algia), *carcinoma* (carcin + oma), and *hematuria* (hemat + uria).

Examples

```
cyst (root): urinary bladder
o (combining vowel): does not add anything to meaning.
scope (suffix): instrument to examine a body organ visually
Cystoscope is an instrument to visually examine the urinary bladder.
```

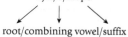

cyst/o/scope

root/combining vowel/suffix

Notice that the combining vowel is omitted because the suffix -ic begins with a vowel as in:

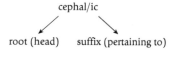

cephal/ic

root (head)   suffix (pertaining to)

Similarly,

aden/itis

root   suffix

In this context, it is worth noting that the combining vowel is retained if a root is added to another root even though the second root begins with a vowel as in:

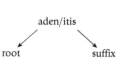

oste /o/ arthr/ itis

root   combining vowel   root   suffix

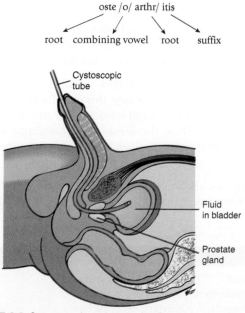

Cystoscopic tube

Fluid in bladder

Prostate gland

FIGURE 1.9 Cystoscope: instrument to visually examine the urinary bladder.

Practice 1.1 Form medical words from the following prefixes, combining forms, and suffixes. Delete unnecessary components.

    a. electr/o/encephal/o/gram _____
    b. enter/o/itis _____
    c. nephr/o/ectomy _____
    d. ophthalm/o/scope _____
    e. trans/urethr/o/al _____
    f. retro/gastr/o/ic _____
    g. bi/o/opsy _____
    h. hyper/thyroid/o/ism _____
    i. arthr/o/algia _____
    j. cerebr/o/vascul/o/ar _____

Reading Medical Terms

Reading a medical term in order to get its meaning is quite easy. You should always start from the end, then move to the beginning, and across the term. A word such as **electr/o/encephal/o/graphy** consists of two roots, two combining vowels and a suffix. We start reading from the last part (-graphy), which means act of recording; then we move to the first part (electr/o), which means electricity; and finally (encephal/o), which means brain. The entire word means the act of recording the electrical activity in the brain.

Notice that if you read medical terms backward, you will change the whole meaning of the term. Consider the meaning of the following two words (reading from the suffix, back to the beginning of the term).

If the word **hemat/o/ur/ia** is read backward, it will mean condition of having urea in the blood, which is wrong because this condition is called **ur/o/em/ia**. Therefore, a medical term has to be read from the end and then to the beginning and across not backward. Thus, the meaning of *hematuria* is a condition of having blood in the urine, whereas *uremia* means a condition of having urea in the blood.

A medical term may not always consist of prefix + root + suffix. In fact, it can be made up of different combinations as shown in the Tables 1.7–1.12:

Table 1.7 Terms Using One Root + Suffix

Root	Suffix	Term	Meaning
ren	-al	renal	pertaining to a kidney
mast	-ectomy	mastectomy	excision of a breast
hepat	-itis	hepatitis	inflammation of the liver
gastr	-ic	gastric	pertaining to the stomach
neur	-algia	neuralgia	condition of having pain in the nerves

Table 1.8 Terms Using One Root + Combining Vowel + Suffix

Root	Combining Vowel	Suffix	Term	Meaning
neur	o	-logy	neurology	study of the nervous system
arthr	o	-scope	arthroscope	instrument to visually examine the joint
bi	o	-opsy	biopsy	removal of a living tissue and viewing it under a microscope
dermat	o	-sis	dermatosis	abnormal condition of the skin
cyst	o	-scopy	cystoscopy	visual examination of the urinary bladder

Table 1.9 Terms Using Root + Combining Vowel (V) + Root + Combining Vowel + Suffix

Root	V	Root	V	Suffix	Term	Meaning
aden	o	carcin	o	-oma	adenocarcinoma	cancerous tumor of a gland
electr	o	encephal	o	-gram	electroencephalogram	record of the electrical activity in the brain
duoden	o	jejun	o	-stomy	duodenojejunostomy	communication between the first and second part of the small intestine (anastomosis)

Table 1.10 Terms Using Root + Combining Vowel + Root + Suffix

Root	Vowel	Root	Suffix	Term	Meaning
oste	o	myel	-itis	osteomyelitis	inflammation of bone and bone marrow
gastr	o	enter	-itis	gastroenteritis	inflammation of the stomach and small intestine
cerebr	o	vascul	-ar	cerebrovascular	pertaining to the blood vessels of the largest part of the brain (cerebrum)

It is worth noting that the combining vowel is retained when a root is added to another root even though the second root starts with a vowel as can be noticed in the examples in Table 1.9.

Table 1.11 Terms Using Prefix + Root + Suffix

Prefix	root	suffix	term	meaning
dys-	enter	-y	dysentery	painful intestine (disorder of a digestive track)
brady-	cardi	-ia	bradycardia	slow heart rate
bi-	later	-al	bilateral	pertaining to both sides
hemi-	gastr	-ectomy	hemigastrectomy	excision of half of the stomach
trans-	derm	-al	transdermal	pertaining to across the skin

Table 1.12 Terms Using Prefix + Root + Combining Vowel (V) + Suffix

Prefix	Root	V	Suffix	Term	Meaning
dys-	men	o	rhea-	dysmenorrhea	painful menstrual flow
a-	men	o	rhea-	amenorrhea	lack of menstrual flow
anti-	bi	o	tic-	antibiotic	substances that are produced outside the body by microorganisms and primitive plants called molds

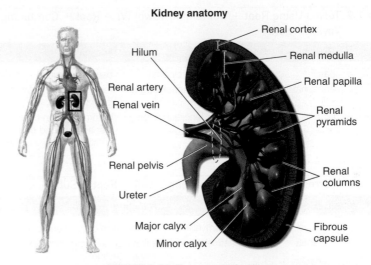

Kidney anatomy

Renal cortex

Hilum

Renal medulla

Renal papilla

Renal artery

Renal vein

Renal pyramids

Renal pelvis

Renal columns

Ureter

Major calyx

Minor calyx

Fibrous capsule

FIGURE 1.10 The anatomy of a kidney.

In conclusion, a medical term may consist of one or more of the preceding combinations. In brief, the major constituents of a medical term are as follows:

1. Root: the part of the term that conveys its basic meaning.
2. Prefix: a letter or a group of letters attached to the beginning of a term to modify its meaning.
3. Suffix: a letter or a group of letters attached to the end of a term to produce a new word form in general or to modify the meaning of the root.
4. Combining form: a root with a combining vowel.
5. Combining vowel: a vowel inserted between a root and a suffix that starts with a consonant or a root and another root to ease pronunciation.

Practice 1.2 Write the medical term for each of the following definitions.

    a. The study of women's diseases is called _____.

    b. Record of electricity in the brain is called _____.

    c. Low level of hormone from a gland in the neck is called _____.

    d. An instrument that examines the patient's eye is called _____

    _____.

    e. Pertaining to behind the stomach _____.

Practice 1.3 Divide the following terms into their component parts and provide the meaning of the whole term.

Medical Term	Prefix	Combining Form 1	Combining Form 2	Suffix	Meaning
gastroenterologist					
hemigastrectomy					
myosarcoma					
antibiotic					
sublingual					
dysuria					
neuralgia					
hypoglycemia					
psychology					
dermatologist					

SPELLING OF MEDICAL TERMS

Correct spelling to writing is as important as correct pronunciation to speaking. Misspelling medical terms may lead to wrong meanings or to life-threatening situations such as death or serious injury to patients. Therefore, it is necessary that you learn the correct spelling of the terms you use in your field. When in doubt about the spelling of a term, you should not hesitate to consult your medical dictionary.

Table 1.13 The "rh" Rule
When a suffix beginning with the letters "rh" is added to a root, the letter "r" is doubled.

Root	Suffix	Term	Meaning
men	rhea-	meno**rr**hea	normal menstrual flow or discharge
hem	rhage-	hemo**rr**hage	excessive bleeding
hemat	rhagia-	hemato**rr**hagia	bursting forth of blood
arteri	rhaphy-	arterio**rr**haphy	suture of an artery
my	rhexis-	myo**rr**hexis	rupture of a muscle

Table 1.14 The "x" Rule

In nouns ending with "x" preceded by a consonant, change the "x" into "g" when you derive an adjective from those nouns, or when a suffix is added to them.

Word	Adjective	Noun	Meaning
larynx	laryn**g**eal	laryn**g**ectomy	excision of the larynx
pharynx	pharyn**g**eal	pharyn**go**tomy	incision of the pharynx
coccyx	coccy**g**eal	coccy**g**es (plural)	tailbone

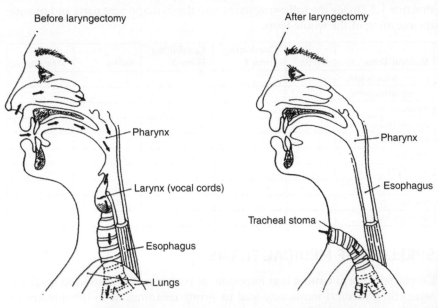

Before laryngectomy

After laryngectomy

Pharynx

Larynx (vocal cords)

Esophagus

Lungs

Pharynx

Esophagus

Tracheal stoma

FIGURE 1.11 Laryngectomy: excision (removal) of the larynx.

When adjectives are derived from nouns ending with "x" that is preceded with a vowel, the "x" is changed into "c."

Word	Adjective	Meaning
cervix	cervical	pertaining to the neck
thorax	thoracic	pertaining to the chest

Basic Medical Terms

The following terms are frequently used in health care fields.

Diagnosis: The act or process of identifying or determining the nature and cause of a disease or injury through evaluation of patient history, examination, and review of laboratory data (state of complete knowledge).

Prognosis: A prediction of the probable course and outcome of a disease (state of prior knowledge).

Sign: Objective evidence of disease or the physical manifestation of injury, illness, or disease. Objective means that the sign can be evaluated or measured by the patient or others.

Symptoms: Subjective evidence of disease or what the patient experiences about the injury; subjective means that it can be evaluated or measured only by the patient.

Syndrome: A group of symptoms and signs that collectively indicate or characterize a disease, psychological disorder, or other abnormal condition.

Acronym: A word formed by combining the initial letters of a multipart name or major parts of a compound term, such as GERD from *Gastro Esophageal Reflux Disease*.

Abbreviation: A shortened form of a word or phrase used chiefly in writing to represent the complete form, such as AMI, for *Acute Myocardial Infarction*.

Eponym: One whose name is or is thought to be the source of the name of something such as a disease, structure, operation, or procedure named for the person who discovered it first, for example, Marfan syndrome, Fallopian tube, Rinne test, Huntington disease.

Acute disease: Rapid, severe, and of relatively short duration.

Chronic disease: Lasting for a long period of time or marked by frequent recurrence, as certain diseases, may be controlled but almost never cured.

Relapse: A return of a disease or its symptoms after partial recovery from it.

Exacerbation: An increase in the severity of the disease or any of its symptoms.

Remission: The period during which the symptoms of a disease abate or subside without having achieved a cure.

Differential diagnosis: The differences between diseases in terms of clinical signs and epidemiological parameters; used as a basis for selecting as a diagnosis the one with the best fit to those seen in the subject. It is also known as to rule out (R/O).

Sarcoma: A cancerous tumor of fleshy tissue.

Carcinoma: A cancerous tumor of epithelial tissue.

Malignant: Tending to become progressively worse and to result in death; having the properties of anaplasia, invasiveness, and metastasis; said of tumors. You can also simply define it by a cancerous tumor that spreads like fire.

Benign: Not malignant; not recurrent; favorable for recovery. You can also define it by a non-cancerous tumor that does not spread.

Myocardial infarction (MI): Death of the cells of an area of the heart muscle as a result of oxygen deprivation, which in turn is caused by obstruction of the blood supply; commonly referred to as a "heart attack."

Cerebrovascular accident (CVA): An abnormal condition of the brain characterized by occlusion by an embolus, thrombus, or cerebrovascular hemorrhage or vasospasm, resulting in ischemia of the brain tissues normally perfused by the damaged vessels, commonly referred to as a "stroke." **Ischemia:** A condition in which blood supply is held back from a part of the body.

Commonly Confused Terms

Many medical terms may look alike because they have similar pronunciation or they may be slightly different in spelling. Students are advised to spell these terms correctly and differentiate between their meanings in order to avoid undesirable consequences.

Examples:

ilium: one of the bones of each half of the pelvis
ileum: third part of the small intestine
intervertebral: pertaining to lying between two vertebrae (intervertebral disc)
intravertebral: situated or occurring within a vertebra (intravertebral vacuum)

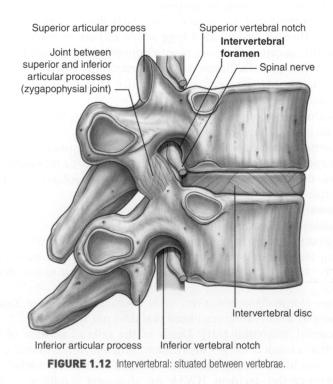

FIGURE 1.12 Intervertebral: situated between vertebrae.

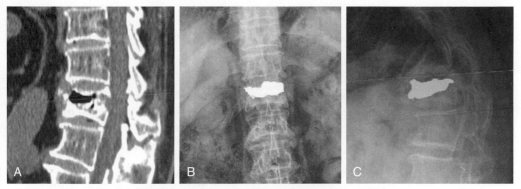

FIGURE 1.13 Images of the spinal column: vacuum cleft.

peritoneum: membrane that surrounds the abdomen and holds the abdominal organs in place
perineum: the area between the anus and the scrotum (or vulva in females)
mucous: (adjective) pertaining to membrane that secretes mucus
mucus: (noun) secretion from mucous membrane
palpation: process of touching and feeling
palpitation: having the heart throb, a feeling that your heart is beating too hard or too fast
albumen: the white of an egg
albumin: protein molecule in the blood
humerus: (noun) bone of upper arm
humorous: (adjective) a general English word that means amusing or funny
humeral: (adjective) pertaining to bone of upper arm
humoral: pertaining to immunity to infection from antibodies in blood
contraction: normal tensing and shortening of muscle from nerve impulse
contracture: abnormal, fixed position of permanently flexed muscle
reflex: involuntary, automatic response of muscular–nervous pathway
reflux: backward flowing of fluid
ureter: (noun) tube that connects kidney to bladder
ureteral: (adjective) ureteral obstruction, ureteral stent, ureteral catheter
urethra: tube that connects bladder to outside of body
urethral: adjective of urethra

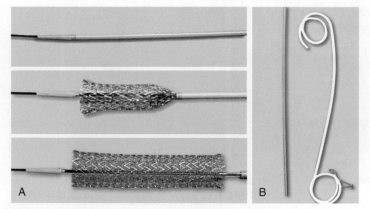

FIGURE 1.14 Ureteral stent: mesh tube that is placed in the ureter to prevent wall collapsing.

vesical: pertaining to the urinary bladder
vesicle: small fluid-filled blister on skin
prostate: gland that surrounds urethra in males
prostrate: lying in a face-down position
breath: (noun) air that flows in and out of lungs
breathe: (verb) action of inhaling and exhaling

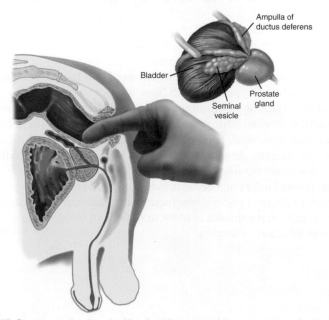

FIGURE 1.15 Prostate exanimation: checking the enlargement of the prostate to confirm benign or malignant tumor.

arteri/o: artery
ather/o: plaque or fatty substance
arthr/o: joint
fissure: groove or crack-like sore of the skin; it also describes normal folds in the contour of the brain
fistula: abnormal passage between two internal organs
infection: the invasion of the body by a pathogenic organism
inflammation: localized response to an injury or destruction of tissues

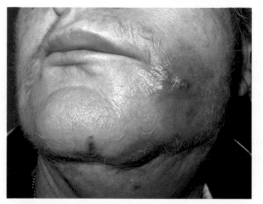

FIGURE 1.16 Infection: the invasion of the body by a pathogenic organism.

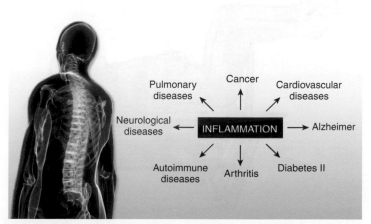

FIGURE 1.17 Inflammation: a localized response to an injury or destruction of tissues.

laceration: torn, ragged wound

lesion: a pathologic change of the tissues to disease or injury

myc/o: fungus

myel/o: bone marrow or spinal cord

my/o: muscle

pyel/o: renal pelvis

py/o: pus

pyr/o: fever or fire

supination: the act of rotating the arm so that the palm of the hand is forward or upward

suppuration: the formation of discharge or pus

trauma: wound or injury

tumor: a swelling of a part of the body caused by an abnormal growth of tissue

viral: pertaining to a virus

virile: possessing masculine traits

Some words are the same in spelling, but have more than one meaning according to the context in which they are used.

Examples

lithotomy: incision to remove the stones from the kidney

lithotomy: an examination position in which the patient is lying on back with the feet and legs raised and supported in stirrups

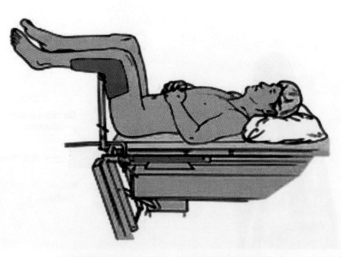

FIGURE 1.18 Lithotomy: an examination position.

calculus: kidney stone
calculus: a name of heel bone
colic: spasm of smooth muscle around ureters and bladder
colic: spasm of smooth muscle around intestines
pelvis: funnel-shaped area in kidney
pelvis: hipbones with sacrum and coccyx
scler: whitening of the eye
scler/o: hardening
myel/o: spinal cord
myel/o: bone marrow
cyst/o: urinary bladder
cyst: filled sac or pouch

PRONUNCIATION OF MEDICAL TERMS

Pronouncing medical terms is rather difficult because many terms are multi-syllabic and some of them have silent letters or have unusual pronunciation. Some differences between spelling and pronunciation are shown in Table 1.15.

Table 1.15 Irregular Spelling and Pronunciation

Spelling	Pronunciation	Example	Meaning
dys	dis	dyspnea	difficulty in breathing
ph	f	pharmacy	a place for dispensing medicine
x	z	xiphoid	cartilage attached to the sternum
ch	k	chronic	pertaining to time (a disease that remains for long period of time)

Table 1.16 Silent Letters

Term	Silent letter/s	Meaning
rhinoplasty	h	plastic repair of the nose
ptosis	p	drooping
pneumonia	p	lung infection
gnathic	g	pertaining to the jaw
psychiatrist	p	specialist in the treatment of the mind
euthanasia	e	painless killing of a patient suffering from an incurable disease

The difficulty in pronouncing medical terms is aggravated by the fact that certain letters have more than one corresponding sound. For example, the letter "c" may be pronounced as "s" that is referred to as the soft "c," or as "k" that is referred to as the hard "c" as can be noticed in Table 1.17.

Table 1.17 Soft and Hard "c"

Soft c (s)	Hard c (k)
cerebral	cardiology
hyperglycemia	arthroscope
encephalogram	cardiac
cytology	gastric
leukocyte	electrical
septicemia	endocrinology
amniocentesis	pericardium
cell	medical
incision	pharmacology

Rule: when the letter "c" is followed by "**i, e,** or **y,**" it is usually pronounced "s"; otherwise it is pronounced "k."

Similarly, the letter "g" also has two different pronunciations. The soft "g" is pronounced "j" as in *large*; whereas the hard "g" is pronounced "g" as in "good" as can be noticed in Table 1.18.

Table 1.18 Soft and Hard "g"

Soft "g" (large)	Hard "g" (egg)
hematology	hypoglycemia
enlargement	electrocardiogram
surgical	organ
salpingitis	malignant
pharyngitis	inguinal
arthralgia	mammography
angioplasty	ligament
meningitis	gallbladder
menorrhagia	gastric

Rule: when the letter "g" is followed by "**i, e,** or **y,**" it is soft "g" as in *large*; otherwise it is hard "g" as in *egg.*

Practice 1.4 Identify whether each of the following words has a soft or hard "c" or "g."

Word	Soft c	Hard c	Soft g	Hard g
esophageal				
esophagus				

Word	Soft c	Hard c	Soft g	Hard g
encephalo				
laryngoscopy				
gallbladder				
cerebral				
sarcoma				
leukocyte				
nephrology				
oncologist				

FOCUS ON READING

Prereading: Answer the following questions.

1. Name some early Arab and Muslim scholars.
2. In which fields did they excel?
3. Select a scholar and prepare a short oral presentation on his achievements.

Read the following passage and answer the questions that follow.

1. Many of us owe more of a debt than we might suspect to the Islamic scientists of the Middle Ages. Muslim chemists, physicians, astronomers, mathematicians, geographers, and others not only kept alive the disciplines of Greek science but also extended their range, laying and strengthening the foundations on which much of modern science is built. Scientific terms with Arabic roots, from algebra to zenith, reflect a period when Islam's activity significantly widened knowledge and ameliorated human suffering.

2. Al-Razi, known in the west by his name Rhazes, one of the most celebrated of Islam's early physicians, lived from 865 to 925. His importance was so great that his colleagues called him "the Experienced." The finest clinician of the age, he has been compared to Hippocrates for his originality in describing diseases. He is said to have written more than 200 books, ranging in subject matter from medicine and alchemy to theology and astronomy. About half the books are on medicine, including a well-known treatise on smallpox. In his discussion of smallpox, Al-Razi was the first to differentiate a specific disease from among many eruptive fevers that attacked man. By giving the clinical symptoms of smallpox, he enabled doctors to diagnose it correctly and to predict the course of the disease.

3. While Al-Razi knew nothing about bacteria, the theory of which was not to be discovered until the early seventeenth century, he had an instinctive sense of hygienic principles far ahead of medieval standards. To appreciate his insights, it must be remembered that he lived in a world where contamination and filth were so common as to go unnoticed, and infections and contagious diseases killed millions. Against this unsanitary

background, he was once asked to choose the site for a new hospital in Baghdad. To do so, he suspended pieces of meat at various points around the city, and at the location where the meat decomposed most slowly, he recommended building the hospital.

4. The high point of Al-Razi's career was an encyclopedia in which he compiled Greek, Syrian, Persian, Hindu, and early Arabic knowledge, as well as anecdotal evidence based on his own extensive clinical experience. This book contributed a great deal to shaping European medicine.

5. Another great Medieval Muslim physician was Ibn Sina, better known in the West by his Latin name, Avicenna. Called "the Prince of Philosophers" by his contemporaries, he is still recognized as one of the great minds of all times. He wrote some 170 books on various subjects and is said to have memorized the entire Qur'an when he was only ten years old. Ibn Sina's most renowned achievement was the *Canon of Medicine*, an encyclopedia that dealt with virtually every phase of the treatment of disease. From the twelfth to the seventeenth centuries, it served as the chief guide to medical science in European universities. Ibn Sina is credited with such personal contributions as recognizing the contagious nature of tuberculosis and describing certain skin diseases and psychological disorders. He also observed that certain diseases can be spread by water and soil, an advanced view for his time.

6. Muslim physicians also helped develop the science of surgery and performed many remarkably complex operations for their time, including brain and blood vessel surgery and operations for cancer. Islamic physicians were especially skilled in treating eye diseases, perhaps because such ailments were so widespread in the Middle East. They wrote textbooks on ophthalmology and invented an ingenious method of operating on soft cataracts of the eye, using a tube to suck out the fluid that filled the capsule of the eye lens.

7. In the treatment of patients in hospitals, Muslims were progressive. As early as the start of the ninth century, there were thirty-four surprisingly modern hospitals throughout the Muslim world. Some of these hospitals had different wards for the treatment of different illnesses. They also had outpatient clinics for the immediate treatment of minor injuries, while patients with more serious complaints were admitted to a ward. In the eleventh century, peripatetic clinics served areas beyond the hospitals' reach. These were moved from place to place on the backs of camels and were generally run by one or more doctors. These mobile clinics were also used in time of epidemics when hospitals were filled to overflowing.

A. Read the following statements and write "T" for true and "F" for false.

1. _____ Al-Razi's encyclopedia had no influence on European medicine.
2. _____ Muslim physicians were able to perform complex operations.
3. _____ Both Al-Razi and Ibn Sina were Latin by birth.
4. _____ Muslim physicians did not know how to perform operations.
5. _____ Muslims had outpatient clinics in the tenth century.

B. Circle the letter of the correct answer.

1. What is an appropriate title for this text?
   a. Mobile clinics in the Middle Ages
   b. The influence of Islamic scientists on modern medicine
   c. Scientific terms with Arabic roots
   d. The clinical symptoms of smallpox

2. In the ninth century, Al-Razi, "the Experienced," was the first to describe specific symptoms of a disease. This was important because doctors could then _____.
   a. write books about it
   b. relate it to many eruptive fevers
   c. diagnose it and predict its course
   d. include them in their dairy

3. Al-Razi wrote an enormous encyclopedia that included medical knowledge from _____.
   a. Greece and India
   b. Persia and Syria
   c. his own clinical observations
   d. all of the above

4. One of Ibn Sina's views that was advanced for his time was that certain diseases _____.
   a. are spread by water and soil
   b. are contagious
   c. can result in loss of weight
   d. cannot be cured

5. Islamic doctors were especially good in the field of _____.
   a. psychiatry
   b. ophthalmology
   c. cardiology
   d. psychology

6. Ninth-century Muslim hospitals were _____.
   a. quite similar in organization to modern ones
   b. quite different in organization from modern ones
   c. simple tents with all patients placed together
   d. nonexistent; doctors made house calls instead

7. In the eleventh century, the Muslim solution to caring for patients in remote areas was _____.
   a. the creation of pharmacies in all small towns and oases
   b. traveling clinics that moved on the backs of camels
   c. an emergency service that brought patients to the doctor's house
   d. hiring doctors forever in those areas

8. The underlined pronoun "They" (paragraph. 7) refers to _____.
   a. patients
   b. Muslim people
   c. hospitals
   d. different wards

9. Find a medical term in the reading text and analyze it into its components _____.

C. **Guessing meaning from context**

Match the words in column A with their appropriate meanings in column B. Write the number of the correct answer next to each word. Base your decisions on the reading passage above.

A	B
a. ameliorated (para. 1) _____ b. predict (para. 2) _____ c. decomposition (para. 3) _____ d. anecdotal (para. 4) _____ e. peripatetic (para.7) _____	1. noticed in personal experience; not researched 2. traveling from place to another 3. to foresee an outcome 4. made better; improved 5. break down of organic matter

D. **Find words in the text that mean:**

1. *A noun* meaning "a subjective indication of a disorder or disease such as pain, nausea or weakness." (para. 2)

   _____

2. *An adjective* meaning "conducive to good health." (para. 3)

   _____

3. *A verb* meaning "to produce (a book, a report, or the like) by collecting information from various sources." (para. 4)

   _____

4. *A noun* meaning "existing, occurring, or living at the same time; belonging to the same time." (para. 5)

   _____

5. *An adverb* meaning "notably or conspicuously unusual; extraordinary." (para. 6)

   _____

6. *A noun* meaning "affecting many persons at the same time, and spreading from person to person in a locality where the disease in not permanently prevalent." (para. 7)

   _____

E. Word building

Complete the following table as required.

Adverb	Adjective	Noun	Verb
_____	_____		analyze
			constitute
	environmental		_____
economically			
_____		establishment	
	evident		_____
_____		distribution	
			create
_____		assumption	

VOCABULARY DEVELOPMENT

Medical Collocations

Practice 1.5 Match the word in column A with its complement in column B. Write the letter of the correct answer on the line provided.

A	B
1. ticklish _____	a. a drug
2. administer _____	b. blood pressure
3. dislocated _____	c. skin
4. sound _____	d. shoulder
5. nutritious _____	e. food
6. weak _____	f. pain
7. sensitive _____	g. advice
8. high _____	h. eyes
9. watery _____	i. heart
10. deep _____	j. cut

Practice 1.6 Complete the following sentences using collocations from Practice 1.5.

1. I fell through a window once and suffered a _____ in my arm.
2. I asked the nurse what to do and she gave me some really _____.
3. I thought I had broken my arm but the X-ray showed I had a _____.
4. My grandfather had a _____ all his life but he still lived into his 90s.
5. The doctor told me I had _____ and should not eat any salty food.

6. I had a _____ in my back. It was the worst pain I had ever experienced.
7. I always eat plenty of fruit and vegetables. It is important to eat _____.
8. The doctor will _____ to the patient.
9. Can we go inside? This wind is giving me _____ and I can't see properly.
10. I have a _____. I always put on sun block cream before I go outside.

Practice 1.7 Match the words in column A with their collocates in column B. Write the right answer next to the correct term in column A.

A	B
1. terminally _____	a. medical attention
2. excruciating _____	b. weight
3. seek _____	c. tooth
4. life _____	d. surgery
5. contract _____	e. consumption
6. regain _____	f. consciousness
7. alcohol _____	g. antibiotic
8. gain _____	h. intervention
9. splitting _____	i. threatening
10. prescribe _____	j. pain
11. surgical _____	k. ill
12. primary _____	l. malaria
13. plastic _____	m. headache

Practice 1.8 Use six collocations from Practice 1.5 and Practice 1.7 in meaningful sentences.

1. _____
2. _____
3. _____
4. _____
5. _____
6. _____

Practice 1.9 What can the following words collocate with?
1. bedside _____
2. gain _____
3. clinical _____
4. biological _____
5. balanced _____

Academic Words

Study the following academic lists.

Academic List 1

Words	Definitions
1. in-depth	covering many or all important points of a subject
2. authority	the power or right to give orders, make decisions, and enforce obedience
3. assess	to evaluate or estimate the nature, ability, or quality of
4. factor	a circumstance, fact, or influence that contributes to a result
5. vary	to differ in size, amount, degree, or nature from something else in the same general class
6. body	the physical structure
7. campaign	work in organized and active way toward a goal
8. derive	to obtain something from a specified source
9. significant	sufficiently great or important to be worthy of attention; noteworthy
10. respond	do something as a reaction to someone or something

Academic List 2

Words	Definitions
1. specifics	concerned specifically with the item or subject named
2. theory	a set of principles on which the practice of an activity is based
3. definition	what is meant by a word, text, concept, or action
4. methodical	done according to a systematic or established procedure
5. requirement	a thing that is compulsory, a necessary condition
6. constituent	a part of a whole
7. data	facts and statistics collected together for a reference or analysis
8. underestimate	estimate something to be less important than it really is
9. contextualize	to place or study in context
10. major	important, serious, or significant

Practice 1.10 Match the words in column A with their definitions in column B by writing the letter of the correct answer next to the word in column A.

A	B
1. authority _____	a. do something as a reaction to someone or something
2. vary _____	b. work in organized and active way toward a goal
3. campaign _____	c. estimate something to be less important than it really is
4. significant _____	d. done according to a systematic or established procedure
5. respond _____	e. being a part of a whole
6. methodical _____	f. the power or right to give orders, make decisions and enforce obedience
7. constituent _____	g. sufficiently great or important to be worthy of attention; noteworthy

A	B
8. contextualize _____	h. to differ in size, amount, degree, or nature from something else in the same general class
9. in-depth _____	i. to place or study in context
10. underestimate _____	j. covering many or all important points of a subject

Practice 1.11 Complete each of the following sentences using the correct word from the box.

in-depth	authority	assess	factors	vary
body	campaign	derive	significant	respond

1. The court held that the Ministry of Health has the _____ to dismiss medical doctors for malfunctions.
2. Scientists made an _____ analysis of the cause of the disease.
3. His most _____ medical achievement was the invention of a new drug for Parkinson disease.
4. I'm going to a _____ concert to support AIDS victims in Africa.
5. The new technique is being tried in medical laboratories to _____ the effects it may have on cancer patients.
6. One of the most important risk _____ for breast cancer is age.
7. Colds do not _____ to antibiotics.
8. The patient's case was very serious. Therefore, it was referred to an expert advisory _____ for further investigation.
9. One can _____ some important conclusions using the results of a proper set of experiments.
10. Medical treatments _____ greatly from state to state.

Practice 1.12 Complete each of the following sentences using the correct word from the box.

specifics	theories	definition	methodical	requirements
constituents	data	underestimate	contextualize	major

1. You have to _____ the remark in the overall discussion to fully understand what was meant in the medical conference about the treatment.
2. We need to draw up some general guidelines for the project before we start getting down to _____.
3. The nurse is very slow and _____ in her work, but she certainly does an excellent job.
4. Breaking medical words into their _____ can help students with the pronunciation of new and difficult words.

5. Well recognized hospitals should establish a method for exchanging _____ for the benefits of their patients.
6. Our hands are recognized by medical professionals as a _____ source for spreading flu and cold germs.
7. Medical researches show that people usually _____ the amount of time it takes them to learn a new habit.
8. Obviously, one of the first _____ to be a medical doctor is that you be in an excellent physical shape.
9. According to anthropologists, there appears to be a universal _____ of human beauty.
10. Current _____ state that some types of cancer could be prevented by taking certain precautions.

FOCUS ON GRAMMAR

Singular and Plural Forms of Medical Terms

Most medical terms are derived from Latin or Greek origins. Most of them maintain their original plural forms, a matter that adds an additional challenge in learning these terms. Fortunately, plurals generally follow some basic rules that enable learners, once they have mastered them, to quickly form proper plurals for most medical terms that they may encounter. However, every rule has its own exceptions. The following are some rules for changing medical terms from singular to plural.

1. **Words ending in "is": change "is" to "es"**

Singular	Plural	Meaning
diagnosis	diagnoses	determination of the cause of the disease (condition of complete knowledge)
analysis	analyses	separation of substances into their component parts
metastasis	metastases	spreading of the cancer
psychosis	psychoses	abnormal condition of the mind
prosthesis	prostheses	artificial part attached to the body

Exception: Sometimes the plural of a word ending in "-is" is formed by dropping the "is" and adding "ides."
Example: "epididymis" becomes "epididymides" (a highly convoluted duct behind the testis, along which sperms pass to the vas deferens)

2. **Words ending in "us": change "us" to "i"**

Singular	Plural	Meaning
calculus	calculi	stone
bronchus	bronchi	bronchial tubes
nucleus	nuclei	nucleus
bacillus	bacilli	rod-shaped bacteria
stimulus	stimuli	something that evokes a response or a reaction

Exceptions

Singular	Plural	Meaning
fetus	fetuses	baby (second month of gestation)
sinus	sinuses	hollow cavity
virus	viruses	an ultramicroscopic infectious agent
viscus	viscera	an internal body organ
corpus	corpora	a dead body

3. Words ending in "ix," "ex": change "ix" or "ex" to "ices"

Singular	Plural	Meaning
apex	apices	pointed ends of an organ
appendix	appendices	a supplementary part of an organ
cortex	cortices	outer part of an organ
varix	varices	swollen veins
matrix	matrices	background substance mold

4. Words ending in "um": change "um" to "a"

Singular	Plural	Meaning
bacterium	bacteria	bacteria
omentum	omenta	abdominal membrane
ovum	ova	egg cells
serum	sera	liquid
ilium	ilia	hip bone

5. Words ending in "a": retain the "a" and add "e"

Singular	Plural	Meaning
vertebra	vertebrae	backbone
conjunctiva	conjunctivae	membrane over the front of the eye
bursa	bursae	sacs of fluid near a joint
patella	patellae	kneecap
pleura	pleurae	one of the two membranes around the lungs

6. Words ending in "oma": retain "oma" and add "ta"

Singular	Plural	Meaning
adenoma	adenomata	benign tumor of a gland
carcinoma	carcinomata	cancerous tumor of a gland
fibroma	fibromata	cancerous tumor of a fibrous tissue
sarcoma	sarcomata	cancerous tumor of a fleshy tissue
angioma	angiomata	a tumor composed chiefly of lymph and blood vessels

7. Words ending in "on": change "on" to "a"

Singular	Plural	Meaning
spermatozoon	spermatozoa	sperm cells
ganglion	ganglia	group of nerve cells
protozoon	protozoa	single-celled animals

8. Words ending in "nx": change "nx" to "nges"

Singular	Plural	Meaning
pharynx	pharynges	throat
larynx	larynges	voice box
phalanx	phalanges	bone of fingers or toes

9. Words ending in "ax": retain the "a," drop the "x" and add "ces"

Singular	Plural	Meaning
thorax	thoraces	chest

10. Words ending in "en": change the "en" to "ina"

Singular	Plural	Meaning
foramen	foramina	opening passageways
lumen	lumina	central opening

11. Words ending in "itis": change the "is" only to "ides"

Singular	Plural	Meaning
meningitis	meningitides	inflammation of the membrane surrounding the brain and spinal cord
arthritis	arthritides	inflammation of the joint

12. The following terms are general exceptions.

Singular	Plural	Meaning
pons	pontes	a band of nerve fibers in the brain
os (mouth)	ora (when referring to mouths)	mouth
os (bone)	ossa (when referring to bones)	a bone (used chiefly in Latin names of individual bones, e.g., *os trapezium*).
femur	femora	thigh bone
paries	parietes	hollow organ
cornu	cornua	• a horn-shaped projection of the thyroid cartilage or of certain bones (such as the hyoid and the coccyx) • either of the two lateral cavities of the uterus, into which the fallopian tubes pass
paries	parietes	a wall of a body part, organ, or cavity, as of the chest or abdomen

In addition to correct spelling, students also need to know how to derive nouns and adjectives from medical terms. Table 1.19 provides examples of suffixes used to derive nouns.

Table 1.19 Noun Forming Suffixes

Suffix	Meaning	Example	Meaning
-ia	condition of	dementia	lack of intellectual development
-ism	state of/condition of	hyperthyroidism	condition of having excessive secretion of the thyroid hormone
-y	condition of	tetany	sustained muscle contraction
-osis	abnormal condition of	psychosis	abnormal condition of the mind
-iasis	abnormal condition of	psoriasis	skin disease
-esis	condition of	diuresis	increased urination
-asis	condition of	menostasis	stoppage of the menstrual flow

Table 1.20 Adjective Forming Suffixes

Suffix	Meaning	Example	Meaning
-ac		cardiac	pertaining to the heart
-ic		metric	pertaining to measurement
-ical		anatomical	pertaining to anatomy
-ar		vascular	pertaining to blood vessels
-ary		dietary	pertaining to the diet
-ory	pertaining to or resembling	respiratory	pertaining to the respiration system
-al		neural	pertaining to the nerve
-ile		febrile	pertaining to fever
-form		epileptiform	pertaining to epilepsy
-ous		cutaneous	pertaining to skin
-oid		lymphoid	pertaining to the lymph

Practice 1.13 Complete the table with the required form.

Noun	Adjective
psychosis	
	abdominal
epilepsy	
	anatomical
biology	
cancer	

Practice 1.14 Write the singular or the plural form as required.

Singular	Plural
bacterium	
	vertebrae
carcinoma	
	testes
ganglion	
	apices
bronchus	
	appendices
foramen	
	larynges

ORAL SKILLS

Students in health care professions need to develop their oral communication skills in order to be able to efficiently communicate with each other and with their patients. Oral presentation skills are essential for professional success. Students need to be trained in how to make effective presentations. When you prepare for an oral presentation, you are supposed to be aware of the following presentation modes:

1. The manuscript delivery
   - Speech is written out word for word on sheets of paper.
   - The language is usually intended to be read rather than listened to.
   - Speaker reads speech word for word with little or no eye contact with the audience.
   - Audience generally loses interest.
2. The memorized delivery
   - Speakers write out a speech (or parts of a speech) and memorize it word for word.
   - Memorized speeches can be effective if the lines are presented the way a good actor would deliver them. However, more often they sound mechanical and stiff.
   - Speakers who rely on memory for their entire speech run the risk of forgetting their lines.
   - It is more practical to memorize short segments of a speech (the introduction, any brief quotes, and the concluding remarks).
3. The impromptu delivery
   - Speaker is generally taken by surprise, has only a few minutes to prepare, and must gather his/her thoughts quickly.
   - Speaker does not usually have notes prepared in advance.
   - Delivery is typically spontaneous and conversational.
   - Speech may seem disorganized, but it can also be very effective.

4. The extemporaneous delivery
   - Speech is carefully planned organized and practiced.
   - Speaker uses an outline which includes main points, key words, phrases, and quotes.
   - Speaker maintains eye contact with the audience.
   - Speaker uses voice expressively, delivering content in a dynamic way.

Presenters should be aware of the following oral presentation skills.

Pre-presentation Skills
General Information
1. Describe the essential components and basic structure of an oral presentation. Prepare an outline for the presentation.
2. Gather information about the topic of the oral presentation.
3. Prioritize the data gathered such that only relevant information is presented and irrelevant information is omitted.
4. Write the presentation in a presentable form.
5. Rehearse the presentation in advance to yourself or to your friends or classmates.
6. Select the relevant visual aids and the relevant technological tools you need in your presentation.

While-presentation Skills
1. Deliver an oral presentation that is stylistically polished and fluent.
2. Avoid reading the presentation as much as possible.
3. Speak clearly and legibly, and pause at important points.
4. Use relevant body language and establish eye-contact with the audience.
5. Inform the audience of the objectives of the presentation.
6. Sum up the main points of your presentation at the end.
7. Make the presentation enjoyable by changing the delivery speed and tone of speech as needed.
8. Speak clearly and loudly enough to be heard by all students.
9. Stand in a position where you can be seen properly, without blocking the chalk board, or the screen.
10. Always keep a hard copy of your presentation. Technology may fail you.
11. Adhere to the time allotted to you and leave a few minutes for discussion.

PREPARE THE INTRODUCTION

Your introduction should have
• An attention getting opener or (hook)
• A preview of the body

A good introduction
• Captures the listeners attention immediately
• Makes them interested in the rest of the speech
• Alerts them to what they can expect to hear in the presentation
• Helps them to follow the information easily

Powerful ways to begin your speech include
• Telling a brief story
• Asking a question to arouse curiosity
• Shocking your audience with a starling quote or fact

POSTURE TALKS.

When giving a speech, here are five ways you can radiate confidence and strength of a character even before you open your mouth.

• Keep your spine straight and rotate your shoulders back.
• Keep your head erect.
• Keep your hands at your sides with your fingers open or slightly curled.
• Keep both feet on the floor and slightly apart.
• If you are using a lectern, be careful not to bend over it or lean on it. Instead, stand naturally erect and gently rest your hands on the sides of the lectern.

Good eye contact.

- Shows that you are open and honest (looking away conveys insincerity/embarrassment)
- Is more effective than the words you say
- Encourages listeners to pay attention to you, to respond to you, and to respect you
- Indicates that you have confidence in yourself and what you are saying
- Allows you to see your listeners' faces to get feedback on how they like your speech
- Allows you to see your listeners' feedback (their nods, gestures, and smiles) let you know that they understand and are interesting in what you are saying

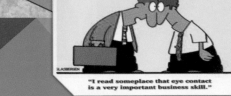

"I read someplace that eye contact is a very important business skill."

EXPLORE BODY LANGUAGE

Experiment with the following body language at home while looking at yourself in a full-length mirror. This practice will help you come aware of how you appear to others when you talk to them.

a. Cover your mouth with your hands while speaking.
b. Sway back and forth on your feet.
c. Cross your hands in front of you.
d. Wrap your hands around your body.
e. Tilt your head.
f. Twirl a stand of hair around your finger.
g. Play with a button or an item of jewelry.
h. Nod your head excessively while speaking.
i. Cross your legs.
j. Look down at your feet.

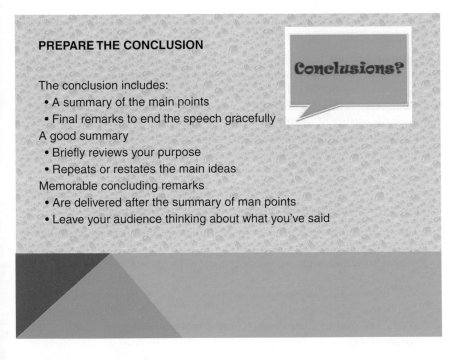

PREPARE THE CONCLUSION

Conclusions?

The conclusion includes:
- A summary of the main points
- Final remarks to end the speech gracefully

A good summary
- Briefly reviews your purpose
- Repeats or restates the main ideas

Memorable concluding remarks
- Are delivered after the summary of man points
- Leave your audience thinking about what you've said

Post-presentation Skills

1. Thank your audience for listening to you.
2. Give them a chance to ask questions or give feedback.
3. Be honest with yourself and audience. If you cannot answer a question, admit it, and promise to look for an answer.

Practice 1.15 Select a topic and start preparing for making an oral presentation. Get the topic approved by your teacher and proceed according to the guidelines mentioned above.

FOCUS ON WRITING

Health care professionals very often need to communicate in writing with each other and with their clients. They need to write the patient's history, physical examination, progress note and discharge summary, research papers, and grant proposals. Unfortunately, many of them encounter difficulty in communicating effectively in writing. Therefore, teaching writing skills should be accorded special attention in medical schools and programs in order to build up the students' writing competence. Each chapter in this book will focus on one writing skill or more. In this chapter, students will be taught how to paraphrase information from different sources.

Paraphrasing means borrowing the ideas of others and putting them in your own words. To paraphrase means to re-write a phrase, a sentence, or more with the same meaning but in different words. The skill of paraphrasing is essential for all language skills: listening, speaking, writing, and reading. Furthermore, it improves the quality of writing, its flow and readability. It also helps the student to understand what he reads before he can convey the ideas of others into his own words. In other words, it improves students' comprehension because they cannot paraphrase without prior understanding of the original text.

In the process of writing, students can benefit from a number of skills and strategies. The following are some essential steps for effective paraphrasing.

1. Read the original text once or twice until you fully grasp its meaning.
2. Write the idea in your own words.
3. Make sure that your paraphrase accurately reflects the meaning of the original.
4. Put the words or phrases that you directly quote in quotation marks in order to avoid plagiarism.
5. Write the author's name, year of publication, and page number of the original text.

Consider the following examples.

a. **Original**: "Paraphrasing is a very important skill for all language skills."
   Paraphrase: Being skillful in paraphrasing is essential for learning listening, speaking, reading, and writing.

   You can clearly notice the difference between the original and the paraphrased version. The word "important" was changed into "essential" and the phrase "language skills" was replaced with four language skills. Furthermore, the word order in the sentence was also changed.

b. **Original passage:**
   "Students frequently overuse direct quotation in taking notes, and as a result they overuse quotations in the final paper. Probably only about 10% of your final manuscript should appear as directly quoted matter. Therefore, you should strive to limit the amount of exact transcribing of source materials while taking notes" (Lester, James D. Writing Research Papers. 2nd ed., 1976: 46–47).

   An acceptable paraphrase:
   In research papers students often quote excessively, failing to keep quoted material down to a desirable level. As the problem usually originates during note taking, it is essential to minimize the material recorded verbatim (Lester, 1976: 46–47).

This is an acceptable paraphrase because:

- The phase "overuse direct quotation" was paraphrased into "quote excessively."
- The original word order was changed. The paraphrase starts with the phrase "In research papers ...."
- The meaning of the second original sentence was restated in the writer's own words.
- The source and the page numbers from which the paraphrase is taken are indicated at the end of the paraphrase.

A plagiarized version:

Students often use too many direct quotations when they take notes, resulting in too many of them in the final research paper. In fact, probably only about 10% of the final copy should consist of directly quoted material. So it is important to limit the amount of source material copied while taking notes.

This version is plagiarized because the same word sequence is used with almost the same words. A few original words were replaced with their synonyms. No citation is given to indicate the source of information.

What techniques can you use in order to paraphrase properly?

1. **Replace some words in the original text with words that have similar meanings** (synonyms). However, be careful. Synonyms do not always have exact meanings. For example, it is acceptable to say "large intestines" but not "big intestines" although "big" and "large" are often given as synonyms.
2. **Change the word order of a sentence** by preposing certain parts and moving others to the end of the sentence. You can, for example, start a sentence with the main clause or the subordinate clause.
   Example:
   a. Students can improve their writing skills if they receive adequate practice.
   b. If students receive adequate practice, they can improve their writing skills.
   You have to make sure that the resulting sentence is grammatically correct.
3. **Change the part of speech of certain words.**
   Example:
   a. The most effective way to become a skillful physician is to receive adequate training on a regular basis.
   b. The most effective way of becoming a skillful physician is receiving adequate training regularly.
   Can you see the changes? Describe the differences between "a" and "b."
4. **Change active voice sentences into passive voice and vice versa.**
   Example:
   a. To become a skillful physician, you must receive adequate training.
   b. To become a skillful physician, you must be trained adequately.

Practice 1.16 Paraphrase the following sentences.

1. The student requested that the professor excuse her absence, but the professor refused.

_____

2. There will be a music concert next to Vienna coffee shop. Would you like to go?

_____

3. International Center is hosting English Conversation classes. They help non-native speakers of English practice their English speaking skills.

_____

4. The office of International Students and Scholars at Purdue University is located in Schleman Hall.

_____

5. The car that was pulled over by the police officer yesterday just had an accident. That driver is not careful.

_____
_____

Practice 1.17 Go back to the reading comprehension passage and paraphrase the following paragraphs.
Paragraph 1

_____
_____
_____

Paragraph 2

_____
_____
_____
_____

PRONUNCIATION EXERCISE

The following are the medical terms introduced in this chapter. You are supposed to read them aloud as many times as you need to master their pronunciation. In this activity, you are also required to give the meaning of each term in order to retain them active in your memory.

Read the following medical terms and find out their meanings.

abdominal
abnormal
adduct
adenectomy
adenocarcinoma
amenorrhea
amniocentesis
analgesia
anemia
anesthetist
angiogram
antenatal
antibiotic
apnea
arteriorrhaphy
arthralgia
arthritis
arthroscope
arthroscopy
autopsy
bilateral
biologist
biopsy
bradycardia
bronchoscopy
carcinoma
cardiac
cardiologist
cardiomegaly
cardiomyopathy
cardiopathy
celiac
cephalic
cerebral
cerebrosclerosis
cerebrovascular
cerebrum
cervical
chronic
coccyges
colonoscopy

colostomy
colposcopy
coronary
cutaneous
cystitis
cystoscopy
cytologist
dermatitis
dermatologist
dermatosis
diagnosis
diameter
diarrhea
duodenojejunostomy
duodenoscope
duodenum
dysentery
dysmenorrheal
dyspnea
dysuria
electrocardiogram
electroencephalogram
electroencephalography
encephalitis
endocrine glands
endocrinologist
endometrium
endoscope
epithelial
erythema
erythrocyte
esophagoscopy
eupnea
euthanasia
exocrine glands
gastric
gastritis
gastroenteritis
gastroenterologist
gastroenterology
gastroscopy

gingivitis
gnathic
gynecologist
gynecology
hematologist
hematoma
hematorrhagia
hematuria
hemigastrectomy
hemiplegia
hemoglobin
hemorrhage
hepatitis
hepatoma
hepatomegaly
hyperglycemia
hypertension
hypoglycemia
hypotension
hypothyroidism
hysterectomy
laparoscope
laparoscopy
laparotomy
laryngectomy
laryngoscopy
leukemia
leukocyte
leukocytosis
macroscopic
mammogram
mammoplasty
mastectomy
megacolon
menorrhea
metric
microtome
multicellular
muscular
myalgia
myoma
myorrhexis

myosarcoma
myositis
myringotomy
nasal
nephrologist
nephroma
neuralgia
neurology
ocular
oncologist
oophorectomy
ophthalmologist
ophthalmoscope
optician
oral
orthopedics
osteoarthritis
osteomyelitis
otalgia
otorhinolaryngology
otoscopy
ovarian cyst
ovariopathy
panplegia
pathologist
pericardium
periosteum
pharyngotomy
phlebitis
phlebotomy
pneumonia
postnatal
prenatal
prodrome
prognosis
pseudoplegia
psychiatrist
psychology
pulmoaortic
pulmonary
quadriplegia
radiotherapy
renal

resection
retrouterine
rhinitis
rhinoplasty
rhinoscopy
sacral
sclerosis
septicemia
sigmoidoscopy
spinal
spondylitis
stenosis
sublingual
tachycardia
thoracic
thoracotomy
thrombosis

tracheologist
tracheostomy
transdermal
transfusion
transurethral
tympanic
unilateral
uremia
urologist
uroscopy
uterine
vascular
venous
vertebral
vesical
xiphoid

REVIEW EXERCISES

A. Determine whether the following statements are true (T) or false (F).

1. A medical term never has more than one root.   _____
2. Some medical terms may not have a combining vowel.   _____
3. Adding a vowel to the word may be necessary to make it easier to pronounce.   _____
4. A vowel must always be present in a combining form.   _____
5. Diagnosis is the complete knowledge of a patient's condition.   _____
6. Autopsy is the examination of a dead body to determine the cause of death.   _____
7. Laparotomy is the removal of the abdomen.   _____
8. Ophthalmoscope is the process of visually examining the eye.   _____

B. Identify the root in each of the following terms and define it.

Term	Root	Meaning of root
1. cardiology	_____	_____
2. gynecologist	_____	_____
3. dermatitis	_____	_____
4. arthroscopy	_____	_____

C. Define the following medical terms.

1. neurology _____
2. gastroenterology _____
3. hematologist _____
4. hepatitis _____
5. gastroscope _____
6. bronchoscopy _____
7. cardiopathy _____
8. gastric _____
9. cephalic _____
10. nephroma _____

D. Spelling: Circle the correctly spelled term.

1.	a. abdomen	b. abdumin	c. abdomin	d. addumen
2.	a. cardiologist	b. cardelogist	c. cardiologest	d. cardeologist
3.	a. resspiratory	b. rispiratory	c. risperatory	d. respiratory
4.	a. artheralgia	b. arthralgia	c. artralgia	d. artharalgia
5.	a. gastro-enterology	b. gastri-centerology	c. gastrio-enterology	d. gastroilogy
6.	a. systoscopy	b. cystoscopy	c. sestoscopy	d. cyctoscopy
7.	a. cardeopathy	b. cardeeopathy	c. cardeopathie	d. cardiopathy
8.	a. diagnosys	b. diagnosis	c. daignosis	d. dyignosis
9.	a. biologest	b. biologist	c. biaologist	d. baiologest
10.	a. excission	b. excicision	c. excision	d. exssion

E. Match the roots in the first column with their meanings in the second one.

1. ren _____	a. to breathe
2. gynec _____	b. kidney
3. ot _____	c. ear
4. thorac _____	d. skull
5. arthr _____	e. hip bone
6. spir _____	f. chest
7. lapar _____	g. skin
8. pelv _____	h. joint
9. tox _____	i. female
10. crani _____	j. abdomen
11. dermat _____	k. brain
12. encephal _____	l. poison

F. **Circle the best answer.**

1. Joint pain is
   a. neural
   b. arthralgia
   c. nueralgia
   d. neuralgia

2. The suffix that means visual examination is
   a. -dys
   b. -dia
   c. -scopy
   d. -ia

3. A malignant tumor of epithelial tissue is
   a. sarcoma
   b. carcinoma
   c. anemia
   d. nephroma

4. The root that means kidney is
   a. pharyngo
   b. rhin
   c. rino
   d. nephr

5. A gastrectomy is a/an
   a. gastric resection
   b. incision of a gland
   c. gastroscopy
   d. examination of the stomach

6. A combining form meaning cells is
   a. cyst/o
   b. cyt/o
   c. cis/o
   d. cyts

7. The suffix meaning "to view" is
   a. -osis
   b. -scope
   c. -opsy
   d. -scopy

8. The suffix that means abnormal condition is
   a. -asis
   b. -esis
   c. -ia
   d. -osis

9. The prefix that means behind is
   a. exo-
   b. dys-
   c. re-
   d. retro-
10. The suffix that means record is
    a. -graph
    b. -ia
    c. -scopy
    d. -gram
11. Tumor of a liver
    a. arthrosis
    b. arthroscope
    c. adenoma
    d. hepatoma
12. Prediction about the outcome of treatment is
    a. prolapse
    b. prognosis
    c. diagnosis
    d. psychosis
13. Which term relates to the neck?
    a. thrombosis
    b. cervical
    c. cephalic
    d. cerebral
14. A white blood cell is a/an
    a. leukocyte
    b. resection
    c. platelet
    d. erythrocyte
15. Subhepatic means
    a. over the liver
    b. below the liver
    c. beside the liver
    d. in the liver
16. An instrument to visually examine the urinary bladder is called a/an
    a. cystoscope
    b. arthroscope
    c. cholecystoscope
    d. gastroscope

17. Low (less than normal) amount of sugar in the blood is called
    a. hyperacidity
    b. hyperthyroidism
    c. hyperglycemia
    d. hypoglycemia
18. Glands that secrete substances are
    a. exocrine
    b. endocrine
    c. adenomas
    d. enteral
19. Cancerous condition of white blood cells with high numbers of immature cells is
    a. osteoma
    b. adenosis
    c. leukemia
    d. anemia
20. Excision of the kidney is
    a. nephrectomy
    b. adenectomy
    c. gastrectomy
    d. mastectomy

G. Identify the suffix in each of the following medical terms and provide its meaning.

	Suffix	Meaning
1. thrombosis:	_____	_____
2. gastrectomy:	_____	_____
3. cerebral:	_____	_____
4. osteitis:	_____	_____
5. retrogastric:	_____	_____
6. carcinoma:	_____	_____

H. Provide the medical terms for the following definitions.

1. _____ : the study of tumors
2. _____ : platelet; clotting cell
3. _____ : pertaining to under the liver
4. _____ : pertaining to through the tube leading from the urinary bladder to the outside of the body
5. _____ : specialist in women's diseases

I. Identify the combining form and give its meaning in the following terms.

	Combining form	Meaning
1. hemoglobin	_____	_____
2. sarcoma	_____	_____
3. prognosis	_____	_____
4. rhinitis	_____	_____
5. transurethral	_____	_____

J. Use the combining forms provided in each question to form medical words.
1. The combining form **cardi/o** to form a word that means a membrane surrounding the heart   _____
2. The combining form **leuk/o** to form a word that means slight increase in normal white blood cells due to infection   _____
3. The combining form **glyc/o** to form a word that means condition of having an excessive amount of sugar in the blood _____
4. The combining form **derm/o** to form a word that means pertaining to through the skin   _____
5. The combining form **gastr/o** to form a word that means study of the stomach and small intestine   _____
6. The combining form **hepat/o** to form a word that means pertaining to under the liver   _____

K. Identify the prefix and give its meaning in each the following terms.

	Prefix	Meaning
1. hyperthyroidisim	_____	_____
2. transhepatic	_____	_____
3. prognosis	_____	_____
4. retrogastric	_____	_____
5. tachycardia	_____	_____
6. hypoglycemia	_____	_____
7. eupnea	_____	_____
8. pericardium	_____	_____

L. Read the following sentences and circle the right answer.
1. If I haven't been examined by a gastroenterologist, I may end up with heavy bleeding, a condition called
   a. hemorrhage
   b. hemoglobin
   c. anemia
   d. uremia
   e. hematuria

2. A patient has had a diagnosis of colon cancer and will need surgical removal of the colon. She will end up with a permanent hole in her abdomen for drainage into a bag. The permanent opening is called a
   a. megacolon
   b. colitis
   c. colonoscopy
   d. colostomy
   e. colectomy

3. You have been having severe pain in your heart, and your family physician refers you to a specialist in the diseases of the heart called a
   a. cardiologist
   b. pulmonologist
   c. neurologist
   d. gastroenterologist
   e. proctologist

4. You have just been diagnosed as having an inflammation of the liver. The doctor describes it as
   a. megacolon
   b. hepatomegaly
   c. macrostomia
   d. hepatitis
   e. gastroenteritis

5. You have taken your son to the emergency room with burning micturition and vomiting. After examination and lab tests, the physician reports that your son has an infection in the urinary bladder and makes a diagnosis of
   a. hepatitis
   b. cystitis
   c. proctitis
   d. nephritis
   e. orchiditis

6. Your sister who is a long distance runner is told by her physician that she has an enlarged heart, but this can be a normal finding in well-conditioned athletes. The doctor writes on his chart that your sister has
   a. hepatomegaly
   b. cardiomegaly
   c. megacolon
   d. macrostomia
   e. myocarditis

7. Your wife is having her uterus surgically removed along with her ovaries. Removal of uterus is called
    a. hysterectomy
    b. orchidectomy
    c. appendectomy
    d. oophorectomy
    e. gastrectomy

8. A male patient complains of having pain in his joints and bones. This may be due to a condition called
    a. endometritis
    b. perimetritis
    c. salpingitis
    d. hepatitis
    e. osteoarthritis

9. A patient with epilepsy has had a procedure performed that records brain electrical activity. This procedure is called
    a. electrocardiography
    b. electroencephalography
    c. electromyography
    d. electrogastrography
    e. electrophoresis

10. A female patient has her breasts removed. The surgical procedure is called a
    a. mammoplasty
    b. mammoplasia
    c. mammography
    d. mastectomy
    e. mammogram

M. **Write the singular or the plural forms as required.**

	Singular	Plural
1.	bursa	
2.		psychoses
3.		bacteria
4.	lipoma	
5.		arthritides
6.	thorax	
7.		foramina
8.	protozoon	
9.		calculi
10.		ova
11.	varix	
12.	meninx	

N. **Circle the correct answer.**

1. Which of the following has a soft "c"?
   a. card
   b. pace
   c. cap
   d. recount
   e. court

2. Which of the following has a hard "g"?
   a. pager
   b. geriatric
   c. genius
   d. good
   e. generate

3. The correct spelling of the adjective for pharynx is
   a. pharnxeal
   b. pharynxic
   c. pharyngeal
   d. phayngel
   e. pharyxial

4. The adjective for thorax is
   a. thoracic
   b. thoragic
   c. thorxic
   d. thorageal
   e. thoraxial

5. The correct spelling for the word that means "a bursting forth of blood" is
   a. hemarrhage
   b. hemeorrhage
   c. hemorage
   d. hemorrahge
   e. hemorrhage

6. The letter "p" in apnea is pronounced as the "p" in
   a. pneumonia
   b. photo
   c. homeopathy
   d. esophagus
   e. phlebotomy

7. A surgery on the nose to repair a postfractured deformity is known as
   a. septoscope
   b. neurectomy
   c. rhinoplasty
   d. cardioplasty
   e. rhinitis

8. The word otorhinolaryngology is made up of
   a. three roots
   b. two prefixes and one root
   c. three roots and one suffix
   d. three prefixes and one root
   e. three roots and one prefix
9. A root with a vowel added to ease pronunciation makes a/an
   a. adverb
   b. combining form
   c. suffix
   d. foreign term
   e. combining vowel
10. Which of the following is a suffix that does not mean condition of, state of, or process
    a. ism
    b. ia
    c. ic
    d. y
    e. sis

Case Reports

A case study report is a document in which doctors describe their experiences in the process of treating a patient. It is a detailed report of the symptoms, signs, diagnosis, treatment, and follow-up of an individual patient. In other words, it is a formal summary of a patient and his illness including the presentation signs, symptoms, treatment, and the outcomes. Case reports may also contain a demographic profile of the patient. Such reports can be shared with other physicians so that they can learn from such experiences. They can also provide teaching materials for students in the various medical fields.

These reports are usually written according to a certain format in order to make them easily accessible to many readers. Prior to writing a case report, you need to prepare the relevant materials necessary for writing the report such as X-ray reports, lab reports, and clinical observations. The case report should only include facts. It should be an honest record of clinical events. Personal impressions and speculations should be avoided. You should also remember that a case report is a record of the patient's progress.

Presenting or writing a case report consists of a number of steps as follows.
1. Provide a context for the case in an introductory sentence:
   This 30-year-old female employee presented for the treatment of recurrent headaches.

2. Describe the complaint, including location, intensity, and associated symptoms:

   Her headaches are primarily in the sub-occipital region, bilaterally but worse on the right. Sometimes there is radiation toward the right temple. She describes the pain as having an intensity of up to 5 out of 10, accompanied by a feeling of tension in the back of the head. When the pain is particularly bad, she feels that her vision is blurred.

3. State the details resulting from the further development of history that pertain to time, circumstances of onset, and the evolution of the complaint:

   This problem began to develop three years ago when she commenced work as a data entry clerk. Her headaches have increased in frequency in the past year, now occurring three to four days per week.

   Describe relieving and aggravating factors, including responses to other treatment, e.g.,

   The pain seems to be worse toward the end of the work day and is aggravated by stress. Aspirin provides some relief. She has not sought any other treatment.

4. Include other health history, if relevant:

   Otherwise the patient reports that she is in good health.

5. Include family history, if relevant, e.g.,

   There is no family history of headaches.

6. Summarize the results of examination, which might include general observation and postural analysis, orthopedic exam, neurological exam, and chiropractic examination (static and motion palpation):

   Examination revealed an otherwise fit-looking young woman with slight anterior carriage of the head. Cervical active ranges of motion were full and painless except for some slight restriction of left lateral bending and rotation of the head to the left. These motions were accompanied by discomfort in the right side of the neck. Cervical compression of the neck in the neutral position did not create discomfort. However, compression of the neck in right rotation and extension produced some right sub-occipital pain. Cranial nerve examination was normal. Upper limb motor, sensory, and reflex functions were normal. With the patient in the supine position, static palpation revealed tender trigger points bilaterally in the cervical musculature and right trapezius. Motion palpation revealed restrictions of right and left rotation in the upper cervical spine, and restriction of left lateral bending in the mid to lower cervical spine. Blood pressure was 110/70. Holding the neck in extension and rotation for 30 seconds did not produce dizziness. There were no carotid bruits.

7. State the final diagnosis:

   The patient was diagnosed with cervicogenic headache due to chronic postural strain.

8. Describe as specifically as possible the treatment provided, including the nature of the treatment, and the frequency and duration of care:
The patient undertook a course of treatment consisting of cervical and upper thoracic spinal manipulation three times per week for two weeks. Manipulation was accompanied by trigger point therapy to the paraspinal muscles and stretching of the upper trapezius. Additionally, advice was provided concerning maintenance of proper posture at work. The patient was also instructed in the use of a cervical pillow.

9. Mention, if possible, the objective measures of the patient's progress:
The patient maintained a headache diary indicating that she had two headaches during the first week of care, and one headache the following week. Furthermore, the intensity of her headaches declined throughout the course of treatment.

10. Describe the resolution of care:
Based on the patient's reported progress during the first two weeks of care, she received additional two treatments in each of the subsequent two weeks. During the last week of care, she experienced no headaches and reported feeling generally more energetic than before commencing care. Following a total of four weeks of care (10 treatments), she was discharged.

O. **Read the following text and answer the questions that follow.**
You are
- a medical assistant employed by Russell Gordon, MD, a primary care physician at Fulwood Medical Center.

Your patient is
- Mrs Connie Bishop, a 55-year-old woman who presents with a swelling in her lower abdomen and shortness of breath. She has no gynecologic or gastroenterologic symptoms. Her previous medical history shows recurrent dermatitis of her hands because a teenager and an arthroscopy for a knee injury at age 40. Physical examination reveals a circular mass 6 inches in diameter in the left lower quadrant of her abdomen. There is no abnormality in her respiratory or cardiovascular systems.

Your role is to maintain her medical record and document her care, assist Dr Gordon during his examinations, explain the examination and treatment procedures to Mrs Bishop and facilitate her referral for specialist care.

1. What type of skin problem has Mrs Bishop had since she was a teenager?

_____

2. She "has no gynecologic or gastroenterologic symptoms."
Define gynecologic. _____
Define gastroenterologic. _____

3. What type of procedure did her knee injury require?
   Describe this procedure._____

4. She shows "no abnormality in her respiratory or cardiovascular systems." Explain this in layman's terms. _____
   To put something in layman's terms means to describe a complex or
   technical issue using words and terms that the average individual
   (someone without professional training in the subject area) can understand, so that they may comprehend the issue to some degree.
   Instead of saying:
   "You need a new piston, valve guides, stator, and counter-shaft bal-
   ancer."
   In layman's terms, you'd say:
   "There are some internal parts that need to be replaced."

5. What symptoms did Mrs Bishop have that brought her to Dr Gordon?
   _____

SELF-ASSESSMENT

Check (✓) what you learned. If you need more information or practice, refer to
the relevant section in the chapter.

( ) I can explain the need for medical terms.
( ) I can define the constituents of medical terms: root, suffix, and prefix.
( ) I can define a combining form.
( ) I can analyze medical terms into their constituents.
( ) I can construct medical terms by applying general rules.
( ) I can use certain medical collocations and academic words properly.
( ) I can pronounce medical terms properly.
( ) I can skim and scan medical texts for main ideas and details.
( ) I can paraphrase a sentence or a paragraph.
( ) I can prepare for an oral presentation.
( ) I can spell and pronounce the new medical terms in the chapter.

CHAPTER 2

Suffixes

LEARNING OUTCOMES

At the end of this chapter, students are expected to be able to:

1. define a suffix
2. identify the functions of suffixes in medical terms
3. pronounce medical terms containing suffixes
4. use suffixes in medical terms
5. analyze medical terms into their components
6. write definitions of medical terms, diseases, and medical procedures
7. use the passive voice properly

CONTENTS

MEDICAL TERMS

It was mentioned earlier in Chapter 1 that medical terms may consist of prefixes, roots, and suffixes. A **suffix** is a letter or a series of letters added to the end of a word to modify its meaning or to produce a new word (part of speech). A suffix, for example, can produce a noun or an adjective. It can also be used to form plurals from singular nouns. Furthermore, a suffix may be used to produce a noun that indicates a medical specialty, a medical specialist, a medical condition or state, a disease, a disorder, a diagnosis, or a procedure.

Suffixes are essential components of medical terms. They are used in decoding the meanings of these terms that can usually be obtained by determining the meaning of the suffix first, to which the meaning of the prefix is added, and finally the meaning of the root.

Combining Forms

The following is a list of some combining forms to which a suffix can be added.

Combining Form	Meaning	Example
abdomin/o	abdomen	abdominal
aden/o	gland	adenoma

Combining Form	Meaning	Example
adenoid/o	adenoid	adenoidectomy
adip/o	fat	adipocyte
adren/o	adrenal gland	adrenaline
albumin/o	protein	albuminuria
alg/o	pain	neuralgia
amni/o	amniotic fluid	amniocentesis
append/o	appendix	appendectomy
arteri/o	artery	arteriorrhaphy
atri/o	atrium, chamber	atriomegaly
axill/o	armpit	axillary
bacteri/o	bacteria	bacteriuria
bi/o	life	biopsy
blephar/o	eyelid	blepharoptosis
brachi/o	arm	brachial
bronch/o	bronchi	bronchoscopy
bucc/o	cheek	buccocclusion
burs/o	pouch	bursitis
celi/o	abdomen	celiac
chem/o	chemical	chemotherapy
chol/o	gall, bile	cholelithotomy
cholecyst/o	gallbladder	cholecystectomy
chondr/o	ribs	hypochondriac
coccyg/o	tailbone	coccygeal
colon/o	colon	colonoscopy
cry/o	cold	cryotherapy
cutane/o	skin	subcutaneous
dactyl/o	finger, toe	dactylospasm
dent/i	tooth	dentist
emphys/o	inflate	emphysema
endocrin/o	endocrine	endocrinology
esthesi/o	sensation	anesthesia
fibr/o	fiber	fibroma
foramin/o	foramen, opening	foramina
gangli/o	knot	ganglionectomy
ger/o	old age	geriatrics
gnath/o	jaw	prognathic
herni/o	hernia	herniotomy
hist/o	tissue	histology
hypn/o	sleep	hypnosis

Combining Form	Meaning	Example
hyster/o	womb, uterus	hysterectomy
ile/o	ileum	jejunoileostomy
isch/o	holding back	ischemia
inguin/o	groin	inguinal
jejun/o	jejunum	duodenojejunostomy
kary/o	nucleus	karyoclasis
lamin/o	piece of backbone	laminectomy
lip/o	fat	lipoma
lumb/o	lumbar region	lumbar
lymphaden/o	lymph node	lymphadenocele
lymphangi/o	lymphatic vessels	lymphangiofibroma
mening/o	meninges	meningitis
men/o	menses	menorrhea
morph/o	form	morphus
myel/o	spinal cord, bone marrow	myelogram
narc/o	unconsciousness, stupor	narcolepsy
necr/o	death	necrosis
noct/i	night	noctalbuminuria
ocul/o	eye	ocular
oophor/o	ovary	oophorectomy
orchi/o	testis	orchialgia
parathyroid/o	parathyroid	parathyroid gland
ped/o	child, foot	pediatrics
pelv/o	hip area	pelvic
peritone/o	peritoneum	peritoneal dialysis
phon/o	sound	phonoscope
phot/o	light	photangiophobia
pleur/o	pleura	pleuritis
pulmon/o	lung	pulmonologist
reticul/o	net/network	reticulocyte
salping/o	fallopian tube	salpingectomy
septic/o	infection	septicemia
somat/o	body	somataesthesis
son/o	sound	ultrasonography
spir/o	breathing	spirometer
splen/o	spleen	splenectomy
spondyl/o	vertebra	spondylitis
tonsill/o	tonsils	tonsillectomy
tympan/o	tympanic membrane	tympanoplasty

SUFFIXES

The following tables indicate the different types of suffixes and their meanings with examples.

Table 2.1 Suffixes for Medical Specialties

Suffix	Meaning	Example	Meaning
-ian	specialist in the field of study	optician	one who makes and fits corrective lenses for the eye
-ist	specialist in the field of study	dermatologist	specialist in the study and treatment of the skin
-iatrics	medical specialty	pediatrics	care and treatment of children
-iatry	medical specialty	podiatry	study and treatment of the foot
-ics	medical specialty	obstetrics	study and treatment of childbirth
-logy	study of	neurology	study of the nervous system

Practice 2.1 Identify the suffix in each of the following terms and write its meaning.

	Suffix	Meaning
1. dermatologist	_____	_____
2. orthopedics	_____	_____
3. physician	_____	_____
4. gynecology	_____	_____
5. psychiatry	_____	_____
6. geriatrics	_____	_____

Table 2.2 Suffixes for Diagnosis

Suffix	Meaning	Example	Meaning
-graph	instrument for recording data	electrocardiograph	instrument used to record the heart's electrical activity
-graphy	act of recording data	echography	recording data obtained by ultrasound
-gram	a record of data	mammogram	record of the breast
-meter	instrument for measuring	thermometer	instrument for measuring temperature
-metry	measurement of	ergometry	measurement of work done
-scope	instrument for visual examination	bronchoscope	instrument for visually examining the bronchial tubes
-scopy	process of visually examining	esophagoscopy	visual examination of the esophagus (food tube)

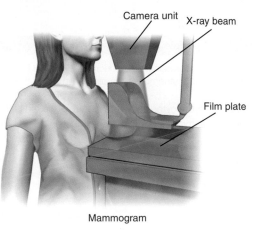

Mammogram

FIGURE 2.1 Mammogram: record of the breast.

Practice 2.2 Match each term in column A with its definition in column B.

A	B
1. microscope _____	a. instrument for recording many physiologic responses simultaneously
2. calorimeter _____	b. visual examination of the abdominal cavity
3. audiometry _____	c. instrument for examining very small objects
4. polygraph _____	d. measurement of hearing
5. celioscopy _____	e. instrument for measuring the caloric energy of food
6. electroencephalogram _____	f. record of the brain's electrical activity
7. echography _____	g. recording data obtained by ultrasound

Table 2.3 Suffixes for the Senses

Suffix	Meaning	Example	Meaning
-esthesia	sensation	dysesthesia	any impairment of the senses
-algesia	pain	analgesia	absence of the sense of pain
-osmia	sense of smell	parosmia	a disorder of the sense of smell
-geusia	sense of taste	ageusia	loss of the sense of taste

Table 2.4 Suffixes for Blood

Suffix	Meaning	Example	Meaning
-emia, -hemia	condition of blood	hypoproteinemia leucocythemia	decreased protein in the blood a disease in which there is a vastly increased number of white blood cells in the blood
-penia	decrease in	erythrocytopenia	deficiency of the red blood cells in the blood
-poiesis	formation, production	erythropoiesis	the production of red blood cells

Practice 2.3 Define the following terms.

1. erythemia _____
2. cytopenia _____
3. hemopoiesis _____
4. calcipenia _____
5. leukopenia _____
6. angiopoiesis _____
7. hepatohemia _____

Table 2.5 Suffixes for Surgical Procedures

Suffix	Meaning	Example	Meaning
-centesis	surgical puncture	thoracentesis	surgical puncture of the chest
-desis	fusion	arthrodesis	fusion of a joint
-ectomy	excision	appendectomy	excision of the appendix
-pexy	surgical fixation	gastropexy	surgical fixation of the stomach
-plasty	surgical repair	rhinoplasty	surgical repair of the nose
-rhaphy	suture	arteriorrhaphy	suture of an artery
-stomy	opening to the outside of the body	tracheostomy	opening of the windpipe to the outside of the body
	communication	colocolostomy	communication between two unconnected parts of the colon
-tome	instrument to incise	microtome	instrument for cutting thin sections of tissue for microscopic study
-tomy	incision	cystotomy	incision of the urinary bladder
-tripsy	crushing	lithotripsy	crushing of stones

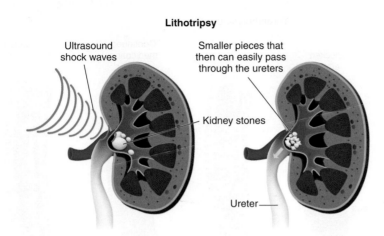

FIGURE 2.2 Lithotripsy: crushing of a stone.

Practice 2.4 The root *hepat/o* means *liver*. Use this root to form a word that means each of the following by adding an appropriate suffix.

1. incision into the liver _____
2. surgical repair of the liver _____
3. surgical fixation of the liver _____
4. excision of liver tissue _____
5. hernia of the liver _____
6. downward displacement of the liver _____

Table 2.6 Suffixes for Drugs

Suffix	Meaning	Example	Meaning
-lytic	dissolving, reducing	thrombolytic	agent that dissolves a blood clot
-mimetic	simulating	sympathomimetic	mimicking the effects of the sympathetic nervous system
-tropic	acting on	psychotropic	acting on the mind

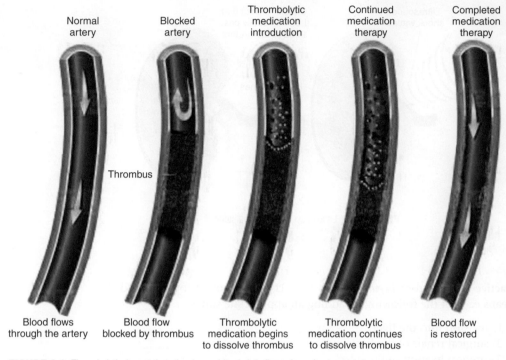

FIGURE 2.3 Thrombolytic (agent that dissolves a blood clot): five enlarged cut-away views of a section of a generic artery with the anterior wall of these vessel segments cut away.

Practice 2.5 Identify the suffix in each of the following terms and write its meaning.

	Suffix	Meaning
1. anxiolytic		
2. chronotropic		
3. parasympathomimetic		
4. somatotropic		
5. neuromimetic		

Causal modeling framework for brain–behaviour relationships in dyslexia

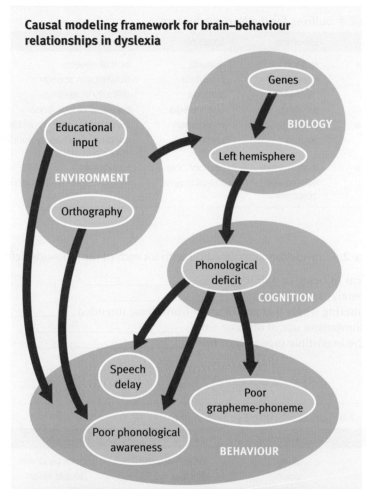

The figure shows the relationship between biological factors mediated by cognitive processes, which affect language and literacy development in dyselxia, and environmental factors, which have an impact at every level.

(Adapted from Morton and Frith, 1995)[5]

FIGURE 2.4 Dyslexia: effects of dyslexia.

Table 2.7 Suffixes for the Nervous System

Suffix	Meaning	Example	Meaning
-phasia	speech	aphasia	lack of speech
-lalia	speech	bradylalia	slowness in speech
-lexia	reading	dyslexia	difficulty in reading
-plegia	paralysis	quadriplegia	paralysis of four limbs
-paresis	partial paralysis	myoparesis	partial paralysis in muscles
-lepsy	seizure	narcolepsy	condition marked by sudden episode of sleep
-phobia	irrational fear	photophobia	fear of light
-mania	excited state, obsession	megalomania	exaggerated self-importance

Practice 2.6 Provide the correct medical term for each of the following definitions.

1. fear of being in public place _____
2. paralysis of the heart _____
3. uttering words that are different from those intended _____
4. compulsive use of obscene words _____
5. the irresistible urge to start fire _____

Table 2.8 Suffixes for the Eye and Vision

Suffix	Meaning	Example	Meaning
-opsia	vision	achromatopsia	color blindness
-opia	vision	diplopia	double vision

Table 2.9 Suffixes for Respiration

Suffix	Meaning	Example	Meaning
-pnea	breathing	dyspnea	difficulty in breathing
-oxia	level of oxygen	anoxia	lack of oxygen in the tissue
-capnia	level of carbon dioxide	eucapnia	normal level of carbon dioxide in the tissue
-phonia	voice	aphonia	lack of voice

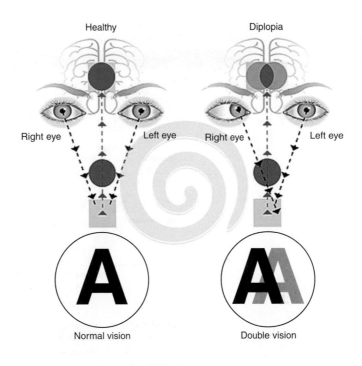

Healthy

Diplopia

Right eye   Left eye   Right eye   Left eye

Normal vision   Double vision

FIGURE 2.5 Diplopia: double vision.

Practice 2.7 Define the following words.

1. eupnea _____

2. normocapnia _____

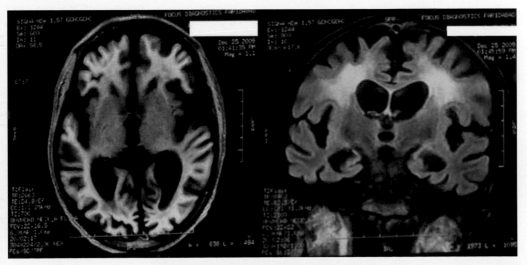

FIGURE 2.6 Anoxia: progressive cerebral atrophy.

Table 2.10 Suffixes for Body Chemistry

Suffix	Meaning	Example	Meaning
-ase	enzyme	amylase	an enzyme that digests starch
-ose	sugar	fructose	fruit sugar

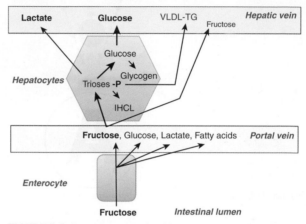

FIGURE 2.7 Fructose: percentage of fructose in fruits and vegetables.

Table 2.11 Suffixes for Diseases

Suffix	Meaning	Example	Meaning
-algia	pain	myalgia	pain in a muscle
-algesia	pain	analgesia	having no sensation
-cele	hernia, localized dilation	hydrocele	local dilation containing fluid
-clasis, -clasia	breaking	osteoclasis	breaking of a bone
-itis	inflammation	encephalitis	inflammation of the brain
-megaly	enlargement	cardiomegaly	enlargement of the heart
-odynia	pain	urodynia	pain on urination
-oma	tumor	melanoma	tumor of pigmented cells
-pathy	disease	nephropathy	any disease of a kidney
-rhage, -rhagia	bursting forth, profuse flow	hemorrhage	bursting forth of blood
		menorrhagia	excessive bleeding during menstruation
-rhea	flow, discharge	pyorrhea	discharge of pus
-rhexis	rupture	hepatorrhexis	rupture of the liver
-schisis	splitting, fissure	thoracoschisis	splitting of the chest

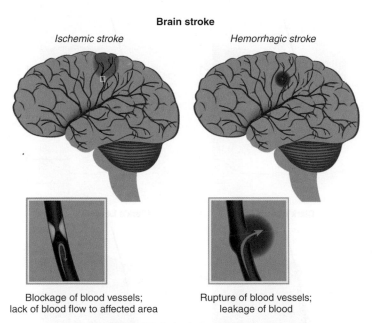

Brain stroke

Ischemic stroke

Hemorrhagic stroke

Blockage of blood vessels;
lack of blood flow to affected area

Rupture of blood vessels;
leakage of blood

FIGURE 2.8 Brain stroke: types of stroke.

Practice 2.8 Match each of the following terms in column A with its definition in column B and write the appropriate letter to the right of the term in column A.

A	B
1. karyoclasis _____	a. having watery stool through the rectum
2. cystitis _____	b. tumor of fat cells
3. gastrocele _____	c. hernia of the stomach
4. hepatomegaly _____	d. condition of having pain in a nerve
5. neuralgia _____	e. breaking of a nucleus
6. adenodynia _____	f. disease of the heart muscle
7. diarrhea _____	g. enlargement of the liver
8. cardiomyopathy _____	h. inflammation of the urinary bladder
9. lipoma _____	i. pain in a gland
10. amniorrhexis _____	j. splitting of the retina
11. retinoschisis _____	k. rupture of the amniotic sac

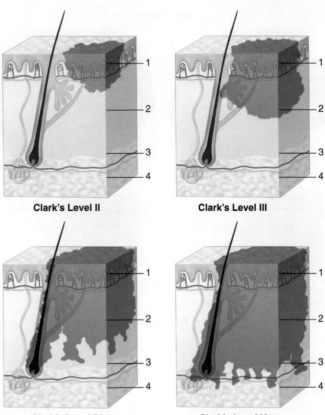

Clark's Level II

Clark's Level III

Clark's Level IV

Clark's Level V

FIGURE 2.9 Melanoma: the four segments of melanoma.

Table 2.12 Words for Diseases Used as Suffixes

Suffix	Meaning	Example	Meaning
-dilation	expansion	vasodilation	widening of the blood vessels
-ectasia	distension, dilation	gastrectasia	dilation of the stomach
-edema	swelling	cephaledema	swelling of the head
-lysis	separation, destruction, dissolving, loosening	myolysis	dissolving of muscle
		hemolysis	destruction of blood cells
-malacia	softening	craniomalacia	softening of the skull
-necrosis	death of tissue	cardionecrosis	death of heart muscle
-ptosis	dropping	splenoptosis	prolapse of the spleen
-sclerosis	hardening	arteriosclerosis	hardening of an artery
-spasm	sudden contraction	bronchospasm	sudden contraction of the bronchial tubes
-stasis	stoppage, suppression	menostasis	stoppage of the menstrual flow
-stenosis	narrowing, constriction	arteriostenosis	narrowing of an artery
-toxin	poison	nephrotoxin	substance harmful to the kidney

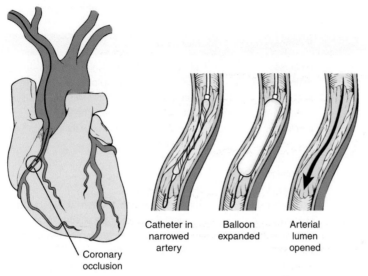

FIGURE 2.10 Angioplasty: nonsurgical treatment of blocked arteries in the legs.

Practice 2.9 The root *arteri/o* means "artery." Define the following words.

1. arteriosclerosis _____
2. arteriostenosis _____
3. arteriospasm_____
4. arteriomalacia_____

The following is a list of suffixes that may not be classified into specific categories.

Table 2.13 Mixed Suffixes

Suffix	Meaning	Example	Meaning
-ad	toward	cephalad	toward the head
-asthenia	weakness	neurasthenia	condition with vague symptoms
-blast	immature	astroblast	immature cell
-cidal	destroying	suicidal	likely to kill oneself
-crine	secreting	endocrine	gland that secretes hormone into the bloodstream
-crit	separate	hematocrit	percentage of volume of a blood sample that is composed of cells
-cyte	cells	thrombocyte	blood platelet
-dipsia	thirst	polydipsia	excessive thirst
-emesis	vomiting	hematemesis	vomiting of blood
-gen	producing	carcinogen	cancer causing agent
-globin	protein	hemoglobin	protein of red blood cells
-kinesia	movement	bradykinesia	decrease in movement

Continued

Table 2.13 Mixed Suffixes—cont'd

Suffix	Meaning	Example	Meaning
-lapse	fall	prolapse	falling forward
-mission	send	remission	lessening of the symptoms of a disease
-mortem	death	postmortem	after death
-opsy	viewing	biopsy	cutting of living tissue to be viewed
-para	bearing	primipara	woman who is giving birth for the first time
-partum	birth	antepartum	before birth
-pepsia	digestion	dyspepsia	impaired digestion
-phagia	eating	polyphagia	excessive eating
-phasia	speech	aphasia	lack of speech
-pheresis	removal	leukapheresis	removal of leukocytes from drawn blood
-phil	attraction	cyanophil	element that turns blue after staining
-phoresis	carrying	electrophoresis	movement of particles into an electric field
-phoria	feeling	euphoria	feeling of well-being
-phrenia	of the mind	schizophrenia	common psychosis
-phylaxis	protection	prophylaxis	prevention of diseases
-physis	growing	epiphysis	part of a long bone growing out of the shaft
-plakia	plaque	leukoplakia	white patch in the mucous membrane
-plasia	formation	dysplasia	abnormal tissue formation
-porosis	lessening in density	osteoporosis	lessening of bone density
-stalsis	contraction	peristalsis	movement of the intestine by contraction and relaxation of its tube
-somnia	sleep	insomnia	lack of sleep
-stat	agent to maintain a state	bacteriostat	agent that inhibits bacterial growth
-tension	pressure	hypertension	high blood pressure
-therapy	treatment	radiotherapy	treatment by using radiation
-thesis	put, place	prosthesis	artificial limbs added to the body
-tic	pertaining to	neoplastic	pertaining to new formation
-um	structure	periosteum	a structure surrounding a bone
-uria	urine condition	pyuria	pus in the urine
-version	turning	retroversion	a turning backward

Practice 2.10 Define the following terms.

1. pericardium _____

2. cryotherapy _____

3. dysphagia _____

4. osteocytes _____

5. exocrine glands _____

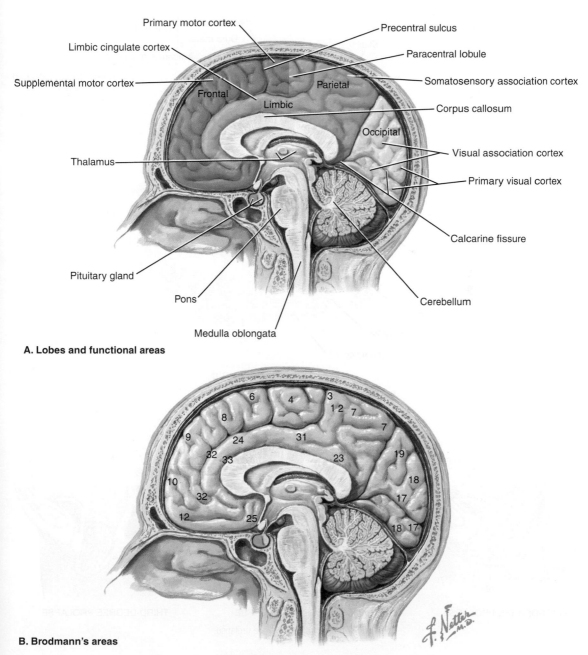

Primary motor cortex
Limbic cingulate cortex
Supplemental motor cortex
Frontal
Limbic
Thalamus
Pituitary gland
Pons
Medulla oblongata

Precentral sulcus
Paracentral lobule
Parietal
Somatosensory association cortex
Corpus callosum
Occipital
Visual association cortex
Primary visual cortex
Calcarine fissure
Cerebellum

A. Lobes and functional areas

6 4 3
8 1 2 7
9 24 31 7
32 33 23 19
10 18
32 17
12 25 18 17

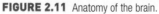

B. Brodmann's areas

FIGURE 2.11 Anatomy of the brain.

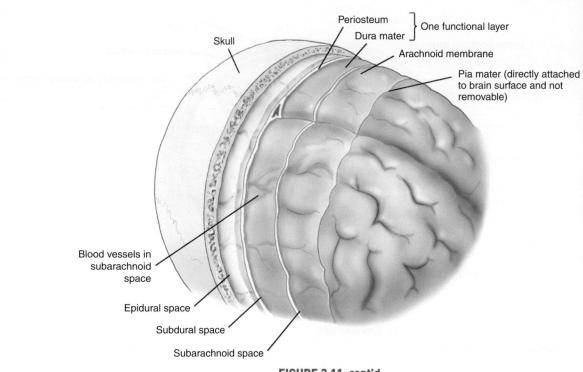

Periosteum
Dura mater } One functional layer

Skull

Arachnoid membrane

Pia mater (directly attached to brain surface and not removable)

Blood vessels in subarachnoid space

Epidural space

Subdural space

Subarachnoid space

FIGURE 2.11, cont'd

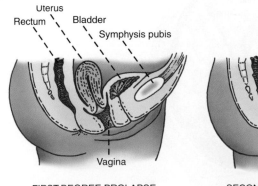
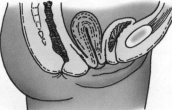
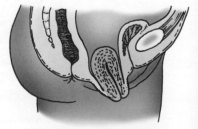

Uterus
Rectum   Bladder
Symphysis pubis

Vagina

FIRST-DEGREE PROLAPSE

SECOND-DEGREE PROLAPSE

THIRD-DEGREE PROLAPSE

FIGURE 2.12 Prolapse: uterine prolapse.

Table 2.14 Terms Using the Suffix -Ectomy (Removal, Excision)

Medical Term	Meaning
appendectomy	excision of the appendix
adenectomy	excision of a gland
hepatectomy	excision of the liver
cholecystectomy	excision of the gallbladder
mastectomy	excision of a breast
hysterectomy	excision of the uterus
oophorectomy	excision of the ovary
laryngectomy	excision of the larynx
nephrectomy	excision of a kidney
colectomy	excision of the large intestine
tonsillectomy	excision of tonsils

Table 2.15 Terms Using the Suffix -Itis (Inflammation)

Medical Term	Meaning
arthritis	inflammation of a joint
neuritis	inflammation of a nerve
esophagitis	inflammation of the esophagus
encephalitis	inflammation of the brain
osteitis	inflammation of bones
dermatitis	inflammation of skin
otitis	inflammation of ears
rhinitis	inflammation of the nose
bronchitis	inflammation of the bronchial tubes
myositis	inflammation of a muscle
phlebitis	inflammation of veins
meningitis	inflammation of the meninges
vasculitis	inflammation of blood vessels

Table 2.16 Terms Using the Suffix -Tomy (Incision, Cutting Into)

Medical Term	Meaning
craniotomy	incision into the skull
laparotomy	incision into the abdomen
thoracotomy	incision into the chest
phlebotomy	incision into the vein

Table 2.17 Terms Using the Suffix -Therapy (Treatment)

Medical Term	Meaning
cryotherapy	treatment using cold temperature
chemotherapy	treatment using drugs
radiotherapy	treatment using radiation

Table 2.18 Terms Using the Suffix -Graphy (Act of Recording Data)

Medical Term	Meaning
electrocardiography	a procedure that records heart wave activity
electroencephalography	a procedure that records brain wave activity
electromyography	a procedure that records muscle activity
angiography	a procedure that records blood vessels wave activity
mammography	a procedure that records breast wave activity
electrocraniography	a procedure that records skull wave activity

Table 2.19 Terms Using Carcinoma (Cancerous Tumor of Epithelial Tissue)

Medical Term	Meaning
basal-cell carcinoma	a slow-growing, locally invasive, but rarely metastasizing neoplasm of the skin derived from basal cells of the epidermis or hair follicles
cervical carcinoma	cancer of the cervix (neck of the uterus)
chondrocarcinoma	a malignant cartilaginous tumor of the epithelium
mammary carcinoma	cancer of the breast
pancreatic carcinoma	the presence of a malignant tumor in the pancreas
osteocarcinoma	the presence of a malignant tumor in bones
colorectal carcinoma	a malignant epithelial tumor arising from the colonic or rectal mucosa

Table 2.20 Terms Using Sarcoma (Cancerous Tumor of Fleshy Tissue)

Medical Term	Meaning
adenomyosarcoma	malignant renal tumor of young children characterized by hypertension and blood in the urine and the presence of a palpable mass
cholangiosarcoma	sarcoma of bile duct origin
esophageal osteosarcoma	cancerous tumor of the esophagus
fibrosarcoma	a form of malignant tumor derived from fibrous connective tissue
osteogenic sarcoma	malignant bone tumor; most common in children and young adults where it tends to affect the femur
chondrosarcoma	a malignant cartilageous tumor that most frequently invades the long bones, pelvis, and the scapula
liposarcoma	a cancerous growth of primitive fat cells
myosarcoma	sarcoma of muscle tissue
Ewing sarcoma	a malignant stem-cell bone tumor, usually occurring in the leg or pelvis of children and young adults
alveolar rhabdomyosarcoma	a highly malignant neoplasm derived from striated muscle
lymphosarcoma	a malignant disease of the lymphoid tissues characterized by proliferation of atypical lymphocytes and their localization in various parts of the body

FOCUS ON READING

Read the following text and answer the questions following it.

Migraine

1. Millions of people all over the world suffer from periodic headaches that can be mild or severe. These headaches are now referred to as migraine. This painful headache may be accompanied or preceded by a number of symptoms, including tingling in the arms and legs, vomiting, nausea, and sensitivity to light and sound. The pain that migraine causes may last for hours, days, or even weeks and it can be moderate or severe in one side of the head. No definite etiology has been reported for such painful headaches.

2. Methods of treating migraine differ from one sufferer to another because different people respond differently to various treatment methods. Some doctors believe that changing lifestyle, getting an adequate amount of sleep, avoiding stress, practicing physical exercises regularly, drinking plenty of water, and avoiding foods that may stimulate headaches may alleviate pain.

3. Research in migraine etiology and treatment has been going on for a long time. Neurologists recently found that a hypersensitive nerve system causes the pain in the head, and they are currently testing new drugs that may suppress the active cells that may lead to headaches. Neurologists believe that these medicines are expected to preclude the painful headaches prior to their occurrence. If they prove to be effective the way they did in the experiments conducted so far, a great number of migraine cases may disappear.

4. David Dodick, the president of the International Headache Society, holds that these medications will revolutionize the methods of migraine treatment. In general, migraine may last from 4 to 72 h. Most migraine patients suffer from periodic attacks during 14 or fewer days a month. However, patients with chronic migraine suffer from headaches for at least 15 days a month. Prior to migraine attacks, it is common for migraine patients to suffer from auras that may be manifest in mood changes, exhaustion, nausea, vomiting, perception of strange light, unpleasant smells, confusing thoughts, or tearful eyes.

5. The symptoms of migraine have been identified a long time ago and different traditional methods of treatment have been tried, including bloodletting (removal of some blood from the vein of a patient as a treatment procedure), trepanning (making a hole in the skull), and cauterization of the scalp. Advances in the treatment of migraine symptoms continued in different parts of the world. At the beginning of the twentieth century, researchers in the field started to examine the role of blood vessels in causing migraine pains, especially after observing the strong pulsing of the temporal arteries in migraine sufferers and the relief they felt after compressing the carotid arteries. Consequently, migraine headaches were primarily attributed to the dilation of the blood vessels of the brain.

6. This belief was later supported by the findings of a paper on the use of ergotamine tartrate. It was found that ergotamine tartrate could constrict blood vessels. Despite the fact that it had some side effects, including vomiting and drug tolerance, it was effective in stopping migraine attacks in some patients.

7. The dilation of the blood vessels (vasodilation) was not the only cause of migraine headaches. It was later discovered that cardiac patients reported that the beta blockers they were advised to take in order to slow down tachycardia reduced the frequency of migraine attacks. Moreover, migraine patients who took medications for epilepsy and depression, and those who used to take Botox injections for cosmetic purposes also reported relief. Therefore, in the treatment of migraines, neurologists started to borrow drugs used in the treatment of other diseases. Unfortunately, the reason why those drugs were partially effective in reducing migraine attacks remained a mystery. Some neurologists believe that those drugs affect various levels of the patient's brain and brain stem in order to alleviate the excitability of the cortex and the pathways that transmit pain.

8. The previous migraine drugs were partially effective and most of them had undesirable side effects. The first specific drugs for the treatment of migraine were the triptans, which were introduced in the 1990s. Richard Lipton, director of the Montefiore Headache Center in New York City, states that these drugs were developed in order to reduce the dilation of the blood vessels that was thought to cause migraine. It was found that the triptans disrupt the transmission of pain through the pain pathways and constricting blood vessels was not necessary to prevent migraine attacks. However, those drugs worked. Lipton added that the triptans were used to prevent migraine attacks and they have become a reliable medication.

9. Some headache specialists like Goadsby, director of the Headache Center at the University of California, San Francisco, are aware of the fact that triptans cannot prevent migraine attacks from happening in the first place. Research that aims at developing effective drugs to prevent migraine attacks is still underway (Adapted from *Scientific American*, November 17, 2015).

A. Circle the letter of the correct answer.
  1. Which of the following best expresses the main idea of the passage?
     a. Migraine attacks affect millions of people worldwide
     b. The drugs used to treat migraine in the twentieth century
     c. The attempts of specialists to develop drugs to treat migraine headaches
     d. The causes of migraine headaches
  2. In paragraph 3 line 5, the underlined word they refers to
     _____
     a. medicines
     b. active cells
     c. painful headaches
     d. neurologists

3. The word "chronic" means _____.
   a. acute
   b. lasting
   c. sporadic
   d. occasional

4. Traditional treatment of migraine involved _____.
   a. removing blood from the vein
   b. trepanning
   c. cauterization
   d. all of the above

5. Chronic migraine patients suffer _____.
   a. from 4 to 72 h
   b. for a maximum of 10 days a month
   c. for at least 15 days
   d. less than patients with sporadic headaches

6. The cause of migraine headache pain in the early twentieth century was attributed to _____.
   a. observation of strong pulsing
   b. blood vessel dilation
   c. compression of carotid arteries
   d. blood vessel constriction

7. The drugs that neurologists "borrowed" for the treatment of migraine headaches were initially prescribed for _____.
   a. rapid heart rate
   b. epilepsy and depression
   c. cosmetic purposes
   d. all of the above

8. Scientists found out that the triptans _____.
   a. disrupt the transmission of pain signals in the brain
   b. constrict blood vessels
   c. entirely prevent migraine attacks
   d. aggravate the dilation of blood vessels

B. Find words in the text that mean:
   1. A noun meaning "expansion, widening." (Para. 5)

   _____ _____

   2. A verb meaning "cause to happen." (Para. 2)

   _____ _____

   3. A verb meaning "occur before." (Para. 1)

   _____ _____

   4. A noun meaning "a warning sensation experienced before an attack of epilepsy or migraine." (Para. 4)

   _____ _____

   5. A verb meaning "caused by." (Para. 5)

   _____ _____

6. A noun meaning "low mood and loss of interest in activity." (Para. 7)

   _____   _____

7. A verb meaning "the opposite of dilate." (Para. 8)

   _____   _____

C. Word building

Complete the following table as required.

Adverb	Adjective	Noun	Verb
x	x		suffer
x			revolutionize
	specific		
x			respond
x			disappear
x			stimulate
x			suppress
x			remove
x		tolerance	

VOCABULARY DEVELOPMENT

Medical Collocations

Practice 2.11 Complete each of the following sentences with an appropriate preposition to form a collocation.

up	down	up	on	of
after	to	about	from	out

1. The patient complained _____ the noise in the ward.
2. She suffers _____ depression.
3. She complained _____ stiffness in the joints.
4. He must have picked _____ the disease when he was traveling in Africa.
5. When we told her that her father was ill, she knocked _____.
6. She broke _____ and cried as she described the symptoms to the doctor.
7. The nurse propped _____ the patient with pillows.
8. The nurses are looking _____ her very well.
9. The workers were exposed _____ dangerous chemicals.
10. They experimented _____ various ways of preventing the disease.

Practice 2.12 Fill in the blanks in the following sentences with appropriate words from the box.

Alzheimer disease	asthma	a cold	ill	serious head injuries
treatment	diet	breast cancer	AIDS	the baby

1. He must know something of dietetics. So, he must have a **balanced** _____.

2. Mariam was **taken** _____ the other day. She's in hospital. They are not sure what it is yet.

3. I got soaking wet and **caught** _____.

4. The health visitor advised the new parents to **burp** _____ after feeding.

5. Ali **contracted** _____while he was working in Africa.

6. As soon as the patient reported severe side effects, the doctor **discontinued** _____.

7. My grandfather **developed** _____ and could no longer remember things or recognize people.

8. He has **suffered from**_____ all his life due to living next to volcanic areas.

9. She had a mammogram and was **diagnosed with** _____ and died a year later.

10. The driver **sustained** _____ in the crash.

Practice 2.13 Match each word in column A with its complement in column B.

A	B
1. detect _____	a. consciousness
2. ease _____	b. the rash
3. check _____	c. the wound
4. adjust _____	d. pathogens
5. inject _____	e. insulin
6. amputate _____	f. the dosage
7. regain _____	g. labor pains
8. probe _____	h. a finger
9. resist _____	i. my pulse
10. soothe _____	j. infection

Practice 2.14 What can the following words collocate with?

1. feel _____
2. insanitary _____
3. sprain _____

4. undergo _____
5. suppress _____
6. incipient _____

Academic Words

Study the following academic words.

Academic List 1

Words	Definitions
1. primary	most important
2. resident	one who lives in a particular place
3. compute	to calculate a result, answer, sum, etc.
4. conduct	to carry out a particular activity or process, especially in order to get information or prove facts
5. administer	to manage, organize, and control something and make sure it is dealt with correctly
6. perceive	to understand or think of something or someone in a particular way
7. restrict	to limit or put controls on the amount, size, or range of something
8. seek	to try to get or achieve something
9. appropriate	suitable for a particular time, situation, or purpose
10. maintain	to make something continue in the same way or at the same standard as before

Academic List 2

Words	Definitions
1. culture	bacteria or cells grown for medical or scientific use; or the process of growing them
2. conclude	to decide that something is true after considering all the information you have
3. resource	something such as a book, film, or picture used by teachers or students to provide information
4. feature	a part of something that you notice because it seems important, interesting, or typical
5. consequence	happening as a result of a particular event or situation
6. positive	a quality or feature that is good or useful
7. affect	to do something that produces an effect or change in something or in someone's situation
8. focus	to give special attention to one particular person or thing, or to make people do this
9. normalize	usual, typical, or expected
10. consume	to buy and use goods, services, energy, or natural materials

Practice 2.15 Match the words in column A with their definitions in column B by writing the letter of the correct answer next to the word in column A.

A	B
1. primary _____	a. happening as a result of a particular event or situation
2. consequence _____	b. to calculate a result, answer, sum, etc.
3. feature _____	c. to make something continue in the same way or at the same standard as before
4. focuses _____	d. suitable for a particular time, situation, or purpose
5. culture_____	e. a part of something that you notice because it seems important, interesting, or typical
6. appropriate _____	f. most important
7. restrict _____	g. to understand or think of something or someone in a particular way
8. perceive _____	h. to give special attention to one particular person or thing, or to make people do this
9. compute _____	i. to limit or put controls on the amount, size, or range of something
10. maintain _____	j. bacteria or cells grown for medical or scientific use, or the process of growing them

Practice 2.16 Complete each of the following sentences using the correct word from the box.

perceived	maintain	restrictions	conducting	residents
administered	primary	seek	appropriate	computes

1. Calcium is the _____ mineral needed for building and maintaining strong bones.
2. Firemen had to evacuate the elderly _____ of a local nursing home after smoke was seen coming from one of the rooms.
3. Our brain _____ millions of bits of information every second of every day.
4. The government is _____ tests of a drug that may prove useful in the fight against AIDS.
5. During the experiment, the drug was _____ to a monkey, and the results were studied.
6. Cigarette smoking is widely _____ as being the most serious health issue in society today.
7. _____ on tobacco advertising and sponsorship are key parts of a global treaty being organized by the World Health Organization to reduce smoking.
8. You should _____ a second opinion if you do not agree with what your doctor said.
9. Studies show that 7 or 8 h of sleep a night is best in order to build, repair, and _____ the immune system.
10. According to a recent study, televised violence suggests young children that aggression is _____ in some situations.

Practice 2.17 Complete each of the following sentences using the correct word from the box.

positive	features	normalizes	concluded	affect
consumption	culture	consequence	focuses	resource

1. The bacteria _____ that we examined under the microscope was actually quite beautiful to look at.
2. The American Psychological Association has _____ that viewing violence on TV promotes aggressive behavior in children.
3. John Kennedy once said that the human mind is our fundamental _____.
4. The sharing of physical _____ by members of the same family creates what we commonly refer to as a family resemblance.
5. Studies show that responses are strengthened when followed by a satisfying _____.
6. Along with a _____ attitude and a healthy diet, your fitness level plays a major role in how you feel.
7. It has now been shown that cigarette smokers _____ the health of those around them even if those people are not smokers themselves.
8. Tonight's program _____ on the difference between human and ape forms of intelligence.
9. Studies show that constant exposure to media content _____ violence, with the result that children come to believe that society is violent.
10. The average daily _____ of salt in this country is much higher than recommended.

FOCUS ON GRAMMAR

The Passive Voice

The passive voice is often used when the doer/performer of the action is unknown, unimportant, or irrelevant to the matter at hand. It is also used when the agent/doer is obvious, and when an impersonal tone is desirable. Passive constructions are frequently used in scientific, technical, and medical texts especially while describing experiments and natural processes or phenomena. This section aims at enhancing the students' awareness of the forms and functions of the passive voice in medical English and research.

Examples

1. The procedure was repeated until there was certainty regarding the results. The problems encountered by the patients were caused by the bacteria.
2. The oxygen-enriched blood is distributed through the cardiovascular system to all tissues.

3. Bones are composed of minerals, organic matter, and water.
4. The protein concentration was determined and the amount of bound protein was quantified.
5. The patient was examined carefully.
6. Twelve hours after admission, a baby was born.

Practice 2.18 Change the following sentences into the passive voice.

1. The skeletal–muscular system supports the body.

_____

2. A tough membrane covers most of the bone surface.

_____

3. The doctor performed an autopsy.

_____

4. **We need the cooperation of several local general practitioners (GPs) to make the new scheme work.**

_____

5. Someone brought this patient to hospital last night.

_____

6. **We can see the beneficial effects of this drug after 1 week's adminis-tration.**

_____

7. Recurrent attacks had troubled Jack throughout his life.

_____

8. The bacteriologist examined the contents of the bottle.

_____

9. People have built robots and used them to make surgical operations.

_____

10. Doctors prescribe certain painkillers to alleviate patients' pains.

_____

Practice 2.19 Write sentences using the passive voice. Start with the following prompts.

1. Vaccines are given to children at an early stage.
2. The laser _____
3. The heart _____
4. The patient _____
5. The nervous system _____

6. Diagnosis _____
7. Viruses _____
8. Medical instruments _____
9. Antibiotic drugs _____
10. The blood pulse _____

Practice 2.20 Read the comprehension passage again and find as many passive sentences as you can. Explain why the passive was used in each.

Practice 2.21 Read the following case report and answer the questions that follow.

CASE REPORT

A woman in her 70s with Type II diabetes mellitus and hypertension presented to a hospital with shortness of breath and was found to have an acute infarction of the anterior wall of her heart. She developed several complications, including renal failure from a combination of cardiogenic shock and toxicity from the dye used for emergency catheterization of her heart.

Hemodialysis was started during hospitalization because of her renal failure. After spending almost a month in the hospital and developing severe deconditioning, she was sent to a subacute rehabilitation facility.

From there, she requested to be transferred to the Mayo Clinic subacute rehabilitation unit, where she spent several weeks. While she was there, she was noted to have symptoms consistent with depression, as well as a prior history of a major depressive episode in 1994. Mirtazapine (Remeron) was started. Mirtazapine is a newer antidepressant, which is structurally unrelated to other classes of antidepressants. The most common side effect is somnolence.

She was eventually transferred to a skilled nursing unit for another month of rehabilitation management of her medical conditions.

At last, she was discharged home to the care for her husband. One month or so after leaving the skilled nursing facility, she came to our outpatient clinic and requested "a top-to-bottom physical."

At that time, she was taking Mirtazapine at 30 mg daily (usual dose 15–45 mg daily) with 11 other medications. She was very focused on trying to figure out a way to recover from her difficulty with walking. She was still participating in cardiac rehabilitation three mornings a week on the same days as receiving hemodialysis.

She scored 13 out of 30 on the Geriatric Depression Scale. A score greater than 10 suggests an increased risk of a major depressive disorder (Yesavage et al., J Psych Res 1982).

On that visit, the medical team focused on the question of whether she would need to stay on hemodialysis long-term and on eliminating unnecessary medications, especially psychotropic medications.

She returned to the clinic, reporting difficulty in breathing and sleeping, fatigue, and poor appetite.

She was felt to have congestive heart failure based on these symptoms. Her hemodialysis regimen was adjusted, and thoracentesis was performed at the request of her cardiologist. Unfortunately, she ended up in a hospital briefly as a result of a fever she had right after the thoracentesis.

On a clinic visit to follow-up on her hospitalization, she looked weaker and was admitted to the hospital for more aggressive treatment of her heart failure. Her dialysis regimen was again adjusted, such that 20 pounds of fluid were removed in the course of the first 10 days. It was also established at that time that she would require hemodialysis for the rest of her life.

When she returned to clinic for her post-discharge appointment, her heart failure seemed compensated and her depressed mood became more evident.

At this time, factors that were possibly contributing to her depressive symptoms included:

1. Medical illness: In this case, her physical disability got complicated by cardiac and renal failure. Other causes such as hypothyroidism were excluded.
2. Other reasons for poor response to treatment were considered. Nonadherence to medication regimen was less likely. Thus, the question of whether the pharmacology of her antidepressant therapy was altered by her renal failure and dialysis became of interest.

Circle the best answer.
1. The -lysis in the word hemodialysis is a
   a. prefix
   b. root
   c. suffix
   d. combining form
2. Which of the following words has a suffix that does not mean *condition of, state of,* or *process*?
   a. rehabilitation
   b. antidepressant
   c. carcinogenic
   d. toxicity

3. The word cardiac refers to
   a. liver
   b. kidney
   c. heart
   d. intestine
4. The adjective pharmacologic is derived from
   a. pharmacy
   b. pharm
   c. pharmacology
   d. pharmacol
5. The suffix in the word "thoracentesis" means
   a. rupture
   b. surgical repair
   c. suture
   d. puncture to drain fluid from
6. "Hypothyroidism" has the suffix
   a. ism
   b. thyroidism
   c. idism
   d. roidism
7. According to the case study, the term for "a sudden and brief but for short duration" is
   a. fatigue
   b. depressive
   c. acute
   d. shock
8. The word "somnolence" in Paragraph 3 means
   a. sleepiness
   b. sleeplessness
   c. depression
   d. complication
9. The word "adherence" in the last paragraph means
   a. treatment
   b. compliance
   c. dialysis
   d. weakness
10. Write a word from the case study that means the same as each of the following.
   a. pertaining to the treatment of old people _____
   b. pertaining to being produced in the heart _____
   c. inserting a hollow tube in the body to diagnose heart disease
      _____
   d. pertaining to having an altering effect on perception or behavior
      _____

11. Find words in the case study that collocate with each of the following words or phrases.
    a. adhere to _____
    b. physical _____
    c. renal _____
    d. side _____
    e. recover _____
    f. admitted to _____
    g. adjust a _____

12. Which of the following term is correctly spelt?
    a. hemodialysise
    b. homeodailysis
    c. humeodialysis
    d. hemodialysis

13. Find a word in the case report that means specialist in a medical field.
    _____

14. In your own words, not using medical terminology, briefly summarize the patient's history.

    _____
    _____
    _____
    _____
    _____

ORAL COMMUNICATION SKILLS

Practice 2.22 Summarize the case study by answering the following questions orally.

1. What is the patient's gender?
2. How old was the patient?
3. What was the patient problem when she presented to hospital?
4. When did the problem start?
5. What were the major symptoms of the patient's problem?
6. What medical procedures were performed to help the patient?
7. Was she prescribed any medicines?
8. Was she required to make any tests?
9. Was the patient discharged or admitted to hospital? Explain why?
10. Why did she need hemodialysis?
11. What happened to her in Mayo Clinic?
12. Name three types of treatment procedures the patient received.
13. What factors contributed to her depressive symptoms?
14. Define the terms: *hemodialysis* and *regimen*.

FOCUS ON WRITING

Definition

Health care professionals often need to define diseases, procedures, diagnostic techniques, or drug administration methods. Definitions can be different kinds. They can be formal or short and informal. For instance, you can give a brief identification of a word's meaning, as dictionaries do. You might offer a synonym. You could say that *significant* means *important* and *shut* means *close*. An informal definition can also use a familiar word or phrase to explain an unfamiliar word or phrase. For example, you could define a *myocardial infarction* as being a *heart attack* and *arthritis* as a *disease*.

A formal definition, on the other hand, follows a three-step method, including the term, its class (the group or category of similar items), and the distinguishing characteristics (the essential qualities that set the term apart from all other terms of the same class).

A chair (term) is a piece of furniture (class) that has a frame, usually made of wood or metal, forming a seat, legs, and backrest, and is used for one person to sit on (distinguishing characteristics).

Arthritis (term) is a disease (class) causing painful inflammation and stiffness of the joints (characteristics).

Practice 2.23 Complete the following chart of formal definitions.

Term	Class	Distinguishing Features
Diabetes mellitus	is a disease	in which body cells fail to use glucose effectively, leading to a range of conditions.
A poison	is a substance	that causes harm or death if it is eaten, drunk, inhaled, or absorbed.
A physician		
An emergency room (ER)		
An (dental) implant		
MRI		

Practice 2.24 How many more general classes can you add to the following list?

tool, instrument, process, procedure, machine, term, piece of equipment, ____

Practice 2.25 Give examples of the following general classes.

feeling: sadness, happiness, anger, etc.
laboratory test: _____
disease: _____
symptoms: _____
vital signs: _____
diagnostic instruments: _____

Guidelines for Writing a Definition

- Avoid circular definitions, or using the term to define itself.
  Do not say: A viral infection is due to a virus attacking an organism.

- Avoid using the phrases "is where" and "is when."
  Do not say: Keyhole surgery is when an endoscope and instruments are inserted through small incisions.

- Do not make your definition so narrow that it excludes facets of your topic. Stating that plagiarism is copying other people's work and claiming it as your own is true, but it excludes other instances of plagiarism.

- When defining a term, start with the material most relevant to identifying the term, rather than saving the best for the last.

- Be as accurate and complete as possible. Avoid irrelevant information. Present ideas clearly and coherently.

- Edit your writing so that errors do not distract the reader, or undermine your ideas.

Practice 2.26 Select a medical term pertaining to diseases, laboratory tests, diagnostic procedures, etc. and write an extended definition for this item.

PRONUNCIATION OF MEDICAL TERMS

The following are the medical terms introduced in this chapter. You are supposed to read them aloud as many times as you need to master their pronunciation. In this activity, you are also required to give the meaning of each term in order to retain them active in your memory.

Read the following medical terms and give their meanings.

abdominal   adenodynia
achromatopsia   adenoidectomy
adenectomy   adenoma

adenomyosarcoma
adipocyte
adrenaline
ageusia
albuminuria
alveolar rhabdomyosarcoma
amniocentesis
amniorrhexis
analgesia
anesthesia
angiography
angiopoiesis
anoxia
antipartum
anxiolytic
aphasia
aphonia
appendectomy
arteriomalacia
arteriorrhaphy
arteriosclerosis
arteriospasm
arteriostenosis
arthritis
arthrodesis
astroblast
atriomegaly
audiometry
axillary
bacteriostat
bacteriuria
basal-cell carcinoma
biopsy
blepharoptosis
brachial
bradykinesia
bradylalia
bronchitis
bronchoscope
bronchoscopy
bronchospasm
buccocclusion
bursitis
calcipenia

calorimeter
carcinogen
carcinoma
cardiomegaly
cardiomyopathy
cardionecrosis
celiac
celioscopy
cephalad
cephaledema
cervical carcinoma
chemotherapy
cholangiosarcoma
cholecystectomy
cholecystogram
chondrocarcinoma
chondrosarcoma
chronotropic
colectomy
colocolostomy
colonoscopy
colorectal carcinoma
craniomalacia
craniotomy
cryotherapy
cyanophil
cystitis
cystotomy
cytopenia
dactylospasm
dentist
dermatitis
dermatologist
diarrhea
diplopia
duodenojejunostomy
dysesthesia
dyslexia
dyspepsia
dysphagia
dysplasia
dyspnea
echography
electromyography

electrocardiograph
electrocardiography
electrocraniography
electroencephalogram
electroencephalography
electrophoresis
emphysema
encephalitis
endocrine
endocrinology
epiphysis
ergometry
erythrocytopenia
erythemia
erythropoiesis
esophageal osteosarcoma
esophagitis
esophagoscopy
eucapnia
euphoria
eupnea
Ewing sarcoma
exocrine glands
fibroma
fibrosarcoma
foramina
fructose
ganglionectomy
gastrectasia
gastrocele
gastropexy
geriatrics
gynecology
hematemesis
hematocrit
hemoglobin
hemopoiesis
hemorrhage,
hepatectomy
Hepatohemia
hepatomegaly
hepatorrhexis
herniotomy
histology

hydrocele
hypertension
hypnosis
hypoproteinemia
hysterectomy
inguinal
insomnia
ischemia
jejunoileostomy
karyoclasis
laminectomy
laparotomy
laryngectomy
leukapheresis
leukopenia
leukoplakia
lipoma
liposarcoma
lithotripsy
lumbar
lymphadenocele
lymphangiofibroma
lymphosarcoma
mammary
mammogram
mammography
mastectomy
megalomania
melanoma
meningitis
menorrhagia
menostasis
microscope
microtome
morphus
myalgia
myelogram
myolysis
hemolysis
myoparesis
myosarcoma
myositis
narcolepsy
necrosis

neoplastic
nephrectomy
nephropathy
nephrotoxin
neuralgia
neurasthenia
neuromimetic
neuritis
neurology
noctalbuminuria
normocapnia
obstetrics
ocular
oophorectomy
optician
orchialgia
orthopedics
osteitis
osteocarcinoma
osteoclasis
osteocyte
osteogenic sarcoma
osteoporosis
otitis
pancreatic carcinoma
parasympathomimetic
parathyroid gland
parosmia
pediatrics
pelvic
pericardium
periosteum
peristalsis
peritoneal dialysis
phlebitis
phlebotomy
phonoscope
photangiophobia
photophobia
pleuritis
podiatry
polydipsia
polygraph

polyphagia
postmortem
primipara
prognathic
prolapse
prophylaxis
prosthesis
psychiatry
psychotropic
pulmonary
pyorrhea
pyuria
quadriplegia
radiotherapy
remission
reticulocyte
retinoschisis
retroversion
rhinitis
rhinoplasty
salpingectomy
schizophrenia
septicemia
somataesthesis
somatotropic
spirometer
splenectomy
splenoptosis
spondylitis
suicidal
sympathomimetic
thermometer
thoracentesis
thoracoschisis
thoracotomy
thrombocyte
thrombolytic
tonsillectomy
tracheostomy
tympanoplasty
urodynia
vasculitis
vasodilation

REVIEW EXERCISES

A. Circle the letter of the correct answer.

1. Inflammation of the brain is
   a. rhinitis   b. pleuritis   c. encephalitis   d. bronchitis

2. The separation of substances into their component parts is
   a. dialysis   b. analysis   c. hemolysis   d. paralysis

3. A benign tumor of muscle is a
   a. myoma   b. myeloma   c. myosarcoma   d. myocardial infarction

4. Enlargement of the liver is
   a. hepatoma   b. hepatomegaly   c. hepatitis   d. hepatorrhaphy

5. An instrument to visually examine the gallbladder is called a/an
   a. cystoscope   b. arthroscopy   c. cholecystoscope   d. gastroscope

6. A suffix meaning a condition of hardening is
   a. -centesis   b. -stomy   c. -plasty   d. -sclerosis

7. Disease of many nerves is called
   a. polyneuropathy   b. neuropolypathy   c. pathypolyneuro   d. polypathy

8. Surgical repair of breast tissue is
   a. mastectomy   b. mastitis   c. mammography   d. mammoplasty

9. Visual examination of the abdomen by making a small incision near the navel is called
   a. laparoscope   b. laparotomy   c. mediastinoscopy   d. laparoscopy

10. Resection of the uterus is termed
    a. oophorectomy   b. hysterectomy   c. urethrectomy   d. salpingectomy

11. The voice box is the
    a. larynx   b. pharynx   c. trachea   d. bronchial tube

12. Ven/o and phleb/o both mean
    a. liver   b. blood   c. kidney   d. vein

13. Prediction about the outcome of treatment
    a. diagnosis   b. thrombosis   c. prognosis   d. psychosis

14. The endocrine gland located at the base of the brain is the
    a. adrenal gland   b. thyroid gland   c. prostate gland   d. pituitary gland

15. Flexible connective tissue found between bones at joints is
    a. skin   b. muscle tissue   c. nervous tissue d. cartilage

16. A vague feeling of bodily discomfort is termed
    a. anorexia   b. antisepsis   c. anesthesia   d. malaise

17. An early symptom of an illness is called
    a. syndrome   b. remission   c. prodrome   d. relapse

18. Which term is not spelled correctly?
    a. retinopathy b. neuralgia   c. electrencepha-   d. vasculitis
                                          logram

19. Surgical repair of the eardrum is called
    a. otoplasty   b. auroplasty   c. somoplasty   d. tympano-
                                                                plasty

20. Eating foods high in cholesterol and fats can cause a collection of fatty
    plaque in arteries. This condition is known as
    a. atelectasis   b. atherosclerosis c. otosclerosis   d. nephrosis

21. Surgical repair of the eyelid is termed
    a. valvulo-   b. acetabulo-   c. blepharo-   d. tympano-
       plasty   plasty   plasty   plasty

22. A specialist of the study of tumor is
    a. oncologist   b. gynecologist   c. pathologist   d. endocrinolo-
                                                               gist

23. What is the combining form for the word "head"?
    a. psycho/o   b. cerebr/o   c. ophthalm/o   d. cephal/o

24. A condition in which blood is held back from an organ is
    a. ischemia   b. uremia   c. hematuria   d. leukemia

25. Condition of having urea in the blood is
    a. leukemia   b. ischemia   c. menorrhea   d. uremia

26. Excessive bleeding during menstruation is
    a. hematology b. hematuria   c. menorrhagia   d. uremia

27. A condition that lasts for a long time is called
    a. acute   b. chronic   c. lateral   d. septic

28. Surgical puncture to remove the fluid from the chest
    a. hysterot-   b. thoracocente- c. oophorectomy d. salpingectomy
       omy   sis

29. Creation of a new opening from the windpipe to the outside of the
    body is
    a. colostomy   b. pharyngotomy c. tracheostomy   d. laparoscopy

30. Pertaining to new development or growth of abnormal tissue is
    a. neoplastic   b. dysplasia   c. hypoplasia   d. hypertrophy

B. Indicate whether the statement is true (T) or false (F).

1. A new connection between two previously unconnected portions of the colon is called colocolostomy.
2. Death of cells is termed as necrosis. _____
3. Subtotal hysterectomy refers to the complete resection of the uterus. _____
4. Osteomyelitis is the inflammation of bone and bone marrow. _____
5. Paralysis of four limbs is paraplegia. _____
6. Treatment by chemicals is radiotherapy. _____
7. Pertaining to under the cartilages of the ribs is hypochondriac. _____
8. Uremia is the abnormal condition of blood in the urine. _____
9. Inflammation of the urinary bladder is cholecystitis. _____
10. Acute appendicitis necessitates appendectomy. _____
11. A specialist in the disease of females is called gynecology. _____
12. Incision of a vein to withdraw blood is called phlebotomy. _____
13. A malignant tumor of epithelial tissues in the body is called adeno-sarcoma. _____
14. Pertaining to the armpit is called axillary. _____
15. A specialist in the administration of agents that cause loss of sensation is termed anesthesiologist. _____
16. Visual examination of what is within an organ is called endoscope. _____
17. An opening in the windpipe is termed pharyngostomy. _____
18. Treatment using chemicals is called chemotherapy. _____

C. Fill in the blanks with the correct medical term.

1. Surgical puncture to remove fluid from the sac surrounding the embryo is _____.
2. Incision of a vein to withdraw blood is _____.
3. Inflammation of the windpipe is called_____.
4. Related to the tailbone of the spinal column is _____.
5. Paralysis of the lower half of the body is _____.
6. A specialist who examines biopsies and dead bodies is called a _____.
7. Abnormal condition of blood clotting is _____.
8. Any disease of a kidney is _____.
9. Pertaining to a blood vessel is _____.
10. Record of the spinal cord is _____.

D. Give the meaning for the underlined term in each of the following sentences.

1. Above 50% of children in the Sultanate are affected by atopic dermatitis.

2. A person with a psychosis loses contact with reality and often shows dramatic changes in behavior. Psychoses can be caused by diseases affecting the brain.

3. A slender endoscope is inserted through an incision in the abdominal wall in order to examine the abdominal organs or to perform minor surgery.

4. A surgical technique for restoring normal blood flow through an artery narrowed or blocked by atherosclerosis, either by inserting a balloon into the narrowed section and inflating it or by using a laser beam.

5. A surgical method of making an opening in the skull; sometimes performed on a fetus during a difficult birth; also called cephalotomy.

6. A procedure for removing metabolic waste products or toxic substances from the bloodstream by dialysis.

7. The surgical procedure of guiding a hollow needle through the abdomen of a pregnant woman into the uterus and withdrawing a sample of amniotic fluid for genetic diagnosis of the fetus.

8. Thoracentesis often provides immediate abatement of symptoms. However, fluid often begins to reaccumulate. A majority of patients will ultimately require additional therapy beyond a simple thoracentesis.

9. A recording of the electrical activity of the brain. It is used to diagnose abnormalities of the brain. The machine used to record an electroencephalogram is called an electroencephalograph.

10. There is a clear difference between a pathologist and a coroner.

E. Give the meaning of each of the following terms.

1. bronchitis _____
2. encephalopathy _____
3. blepharoptosis _____
4. tympanoplasty _____
5. necrosis _____
6. hysterectomy _____
7. colonoscopy _____
8. neuralgia _____
9. celiac _____
10. craniotomy _____
11. subcutaneous _____
12. jejunoileostomy _____
13. phonoscope _____
14. ultrasonography _____
15. dermatologist _____

F. Give the meaning of each of the following suffixes.

1. -pathy_____
2. -iatry_____
3. -ics_____
4. -gram_____
5. -meter_____
6. -osis_____
7. -ical_____
8. -ectomy_____
9. -rhaphy _____
10. -centesis _____
11. -logist _____
12. -sclerosis_____
13. -ptosis _____
14. -toxin _____
15. -cele _____
16. -rhagia _____
17. -odynia _____
18. -megaly _____
19. -edema _____
20. -tripsy _____

G. Circle the correct answer.

1. The suffix in the word insomnia is
   a. in
   b. nia
   c. a
   d. ia
2. The suffix in sclerosis is
   a. sis
   b. ros
   c. scler
   d. is
3. The adjective suffix in febrile is
   a. e
   b. le
   c. ile
   d. brile
4. Cytogenesis is
   a. formation of cells
   b. division of the nucleus
   c. formation of proteins
   d. formation of fibers

5. A megakaryocyte is a cell with a large
   a. membrane
   b. nucleus
   c. cytoplasm
   d. wall
6. A histologist studies
   a. genetics
   b. surgery
   c. chemistry
   d. tissues
7. A fibroadenoma is a fibrous tumor of
   a. muscle
   b. gland
   c. heart
   d. skull
8. In adiposuria, the urine contains
   a. sugar
   b. carbohydrate
   c. protein
   d. fat
9. Macrosomia refers to a large
   a. tooth
   b. gland
   c. body
   d. nucleus
10. The suffix -ase indicates a/an
   a. sugar
   b. starch
   c. cell
   d. enzyme
11. A lipase is
   a. a carbohydrate that digests fat
   b. a fat that digests carbohydrates
   c. an enzyme that digests fats
   d. a protein that digests cartilage
12. Death of tissue is termed
   a. bruising
   b. bleeding
   c. rupture
   d. necrosis
13. A toxin is a
   a. fever
   b. drug
   c. poison
   d. test

14. A cancer of muscle or connective tissue is termed
    a. epithelioma
    b. carcinoma
    c. leukemia
    d. sarcoma
15. A hernia is
    a. death of an organ
    b. protrusion of an organ through an abnormal opening
    c. constriction of a vessel or organ
    d. twisting of a channel
16. Sepsis is caused by
    a. fever
    b. inflammation
    c. bleeding
    d. microorganisms
17. Adenopathy is
    a. inflammation of a muscle
    b. any disease of the lungs
    c. enlargement of a gland
    d. any disease of a gland
18. Arteriosclerosis is
    a. softening of the arteries
    b. widening of the veins
    c. hardening of the arteries
    d. narrowing of the vessels
19. Pain in the stomach is
    a. gastrostenosis
    b. gastropyretic
    c. gastrolithiasis
    d. gastralgia
20. In osteoclasis, a bone is
    a. bent
    b. arthritic
    c. broken
    d. disjointed
21. The suffix -odynia means the same as
    a. oma
    b. itis
    c. rhagia
    d. algia
22. The term hepatorrhexis describes
    a. dropping of the liver
    b. enlargement of the liver
    c. softening of the liver
    d. rupture of the liver

23. The suffix in seborrhea means
    a. discharge
    b. blockage
    c. thinning
    d. infection
24. In retinoschisis, the retina of the eye is
    a. dislocated
    b. split
    c. healed
    d. thickened
25. A word that means enlargement of the spleen is
    a. splenomegaly
    b. splenopathy
    c. splenitis
    d. splenorrhagia
26. Hepatomalacia is
    a. hardening of the liver
    b. softening of the liver
    c. rupture of the spleen
    d. hemorrhage of the liver
27. Tracheostenosis is
    a. widening of the trachea
    b. rupture of the windpipe
    c. narrowing of the throat
    d. narrowing of the trachea
28. A word that means separation, dissolving, destruction is
    a. ptosis
    b. ectasia
    c. stasis
    d. lysis
29. A word for swelling caused by accumulation of fluid is
    a. malacia
    b. stenosis
    c. edema
    d. spasm
30. A synonym for dilatation is
    a. lithiasis
    b. exacerbation
    c. necrosis
    d. ectasia

31. In blepharoptosis, the eyelids
    a. thin
    b. separate
    c. harden
    d. droop
32. The word stasis means
    a. profuse flow
    b. spasm
    c. swelling
    d. stoppage
33. Cryotherapy is treatment with
    a. drugs
    b. heat
    c. cold
    d. radiation
34. A phonostethograph
    a. records heat waves
    b. measures energy
    c. releases air
    d. records chest sounds
35. A calorimeter
    a. measures calories
    b. generates heat
    c. generates calories
    d. is used to inspect internal organs
36. A radiograph is made with
    a. light
    b. heat
    c. sound
    d. X-rays
37. Laparoscopy is
    a. suture of the abdomen
    b. examination of the abdomen
    c. recording of abdominal sounds
    d. examination of the throat
38. Binding of pleural membranes is called
    a. pleurodesis
    b. pleurectomy
    c. pleurometry
    d. pleurocentesis

39. Lithotripsy is
    a. measurement of calculi
    b. surgical removal of a stone
    c. crushing of a stone
    d. removal of calculi
40. Arthroplasty is
    a. measurement of a joint
    b. fusion of a joint
    c. surgery on the ear
    d. plastic repair of a joint
41. In gastropexy, the stomach is
    a. widened
    b. surgically fixed
    c. dilated
    d. stapled for weight loss
42. In a hepatorrhaphy, the liver is
    a. divided
    b. drained
    c. stained
    d. repaired
43. The ending in the word sympathomimetic means
    a. enhancing
    b. counteracting
    c. simulating
    d. ending
44. A hypnotic drug is one that
    a. maintains wakefulness
    b. reduces allergic responses
    c. induces sleep
    d. stimulates nervous activity in the body
45. Cardioptosis is
    a. downward displacement of the heart
    b. irregularity of the heartbeat
    c. rupture of the heart
    d. cardiomyopathy
46. A valvotome is a/an
    a. flap of a valve
    b. instrument for incising a valve
    c. instrument for measuring a valve
    d. cusp of a valve
47. Phlebectasia is
    a. constriction of a vein
    b. spasm of a vein
    c. dilatation of a capillary
    d. dilatation of a vein

48. Arteriostenosis is
    a. widening of an artery
    b. growth of an artery
    c. shrinking of an arteriole
    d. narrowing of an artery
49. A lymphangioma is a/an
    a. tumor of lymph nodes
    b. inflammation of lymphatic vessels
    c. tumor of lymphatic vessels
    d. removal of lymph nodes
50. Cytopenia is a/an
    a. deficiency of cells
    b. excess of cells
    c. distorted shape of cells
    d. enlargement of cells
51. Erythropoiesis is
    a. formation of white cells
    b. formation of red cells
    c. destruction of red cells
    d. formation of platelets
52. The root in ischemia means
    a. holding back
    b. chemical
    c. chemistry
    d. lack of
53. Lymphopoiesis is
    a. formation of lymph
    b. formation of lymphocytes
    c. destruction of lymphocytes
    d. formation of macrophages
54. Thrombolysis is
    a. destruction of a blood clot
    b. measurement of clotting time
    c. formation of a blood clot
    d. formation of platelets
55. A cystocele is a
    a. dilatation of the bladder
    b. shrinking of the bladder
    c. dropping of the bladder
    d. hernia of the bladder

SELF-ASSESSMENT

Check (✓) what you learned. If you need more information or practice, refer to the relevant section in the chapter.

( ) I can define a suffix.
( ) I can identify suffixes in medical terms.
( ) I can differentiate between the suffixes that have the same function.
( ) I can analyze medical terms into their constituents.
( ) I can use suffixes in medical terms.
( ) I can use certain medical collocations and academic words properly.
( ) I can pronounce medical terms properly.
( ) I can read medical texts for main ideas and details.
( ) I can ask and answer questions pertaining to medical issues.
( ) I can report medical cases orally.
( ) I can spell the new medical terms in the chapter.

Prefixes

CONTENTS

MEDICAL TERMS

A prefix is a letter or a group of letters attached to the beginning of a word to modify or change its meaning. Pre- in the word "prefix" means before. Prefixes are common components of medical terms. They may indicate location, number, time, color, and opposite meanings, etc. Prefixes are never used independently. They have to be added to the beginning of words with a hyphen. However, medical dictionaries nowadays drop the hyphen after many frequent prefixes. They can be added before verbs, nouns, and adjectives to modify their meanings. Learning prefixes is essential to health care students because they are frequently used in building up medical terminology. Furthermore, they are necessary for understanding the meanings of medical terms. Most of the medical prefixes come from Latin or Greek origins and that is why they are commonly used in the international language of science and medicine.

Consider the following examples and note the different meaning that results when a new prefix is added to the same root.

Prefix	Medical Term	Meaning
hypo- (beneath or below)	hypothyroidism	abnormally low activity of the thyroid gland
hyper- (over)	hyperthyroidism	overactivity of the thyroid gland

Prefix	Medical Term	Meaning
a- (lack of)	apnea	cessation of breathing
dys- (difficulty)	dyspnea	difficulty in breathing
bi- (two)	bilateral	pertaining to two sides
uni- (one)	unilateral	pertaining to one side

Combining Forms

The following is a list of some combining forms to which a prefix can be added:

Combining Form	Meaning	Example
an/o	anus	perianal
carp/o	wrist bone	metacarpal
cis/o	cutting	incision
cost/o	ribs	subcostal
crani/o	skull	extracranial
crin/o	secretion	endocrine
dactyl/o	fingers or toes	polydactyly
dur/o	dura mater	subdural hematoma
gen/o	produce	congenital
ign/o	fire	malignant
later/o	side	bilateral
lingu/o	tongue	sublingual
nat/i	birth	postnatal
norm/o	rule/order	abnormal
peritone/o	peritoneum	retroperitoneal
phag/o	appetite	polyphagia
phas/o	speech	aphasia
plas/o	formation	dysplasia
pleg/o	paralysis	quadriplegia
scapul/o	shoulder blades	subscapular
sect/o	cutting	resection
thyroid/o	thyroid hormone	hyperthyroidism
top/o	to put/place	ectopic
troph/o	development	atrophy
urethr/o	urethra	transurethral
uter/o	uterus	intrauterine
ven/o	vein	intravenous
vertebr/o	backbone	intervertebral

PREFIXES

The following tables display the different types of prefixes and their meanings with examples.

Table 3.1 Prefixes for Direction

Prefix	Meaning	Example	Meaning
ab-	away from	abduct	to move away from the midline
ad-	toward	adjacent	being near or close
dia-	through	diameter	through measurement
trans-	through	transdermal	pertaining to through the skin
per-	through	permeable	capable of being penetrated by liquids or gases

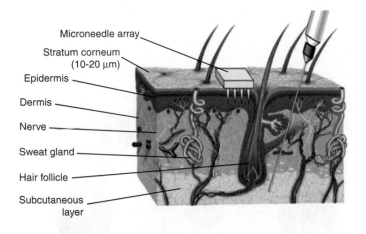

Microneedle array
Stratum corneum
(10-20 µm)
Epidermis
Dermis
Nerve
Sweat gland
Hair follicle
Subcutaneous
layer

FIGURE 3.1 Transdermal: pertaining to through the skin.

Practice 3.1 Identify the prefix in each of the following words and write its meaning.

Prefix	Meaning
1. adduct _____	_____
2. percolate _____	_____
3. dialysis _____	_____
4. adhere _____	_____
5. transurethral _____	_____
6. abnormal _____	_____

Table 3.2 Prefixes for Numbers

Prefix	Meaning	Example	Meaning
prim/i-	first	primitive, primary	occurring first in time or sequence
mon/o-	one	monocular	a microscope with one lens
uni-	one	unilateral	one side
hemi-	half	hemiplegia	one side paralysis
semi-	half	semilunar	shaped like a half moon
bi-	two	bipolar	having two poles
di-	two	diatomic	having two atoms
dipl/o-	double	diplopic	pertaining to double vision
tri-	three	tripod	having three legs
quadri-	four	quadriplegia	paralysis of four limbs
tetra-	four	tetrad	four components
multi-	many	multicellular	consisting of many cells
poly-	many	polyphagia	excessive appetite

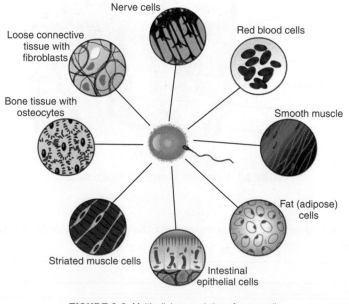

FIGURE 3.2 Multicellular: consisting of many cells.

Practice 3.2 Match each term in column A with its meaning in column B.

A	B
1. diploid	a. an element that has one atom
2. polyneuropathy	b. half solid
3. monoatomic	c. disease of many nerves
4. unify	d. make two or more in one parts
5. semisolid	e. an organism that has two sets of chromosome

Table 3.3 Prefixes for Colors

Prefix	Meaning	Example	Meaning
leuk/o-	white	leukoplakia	having white patches in the mouth
cyan/o-	blue	cyanosis	bluish discoloration of the skin
erythr/o-	red	erythrocyte	red blood cell
melan/o-	black, dark	melanin	the dark pigment that colors the hair and skin
poli/o-	gray	poliomyelitis	inflammation of the gray matter of the brain
xanth/o-	yellow	xanthoderma	yellow coloration of the skin

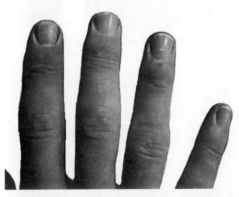

FIGURE 3.3 Cyanosis: bluish discoloration of the skin.

Practice 3.3 Define the following terms.

1. leukemia _____
2. xanthoma _____
3. melanocyte _____
4. erythrocytosis _____

Table 3.4 Prefixes for Time or Position

Prefix	Meaning	Example	Meaning
ante-	before	antepartum	before birth
pre-	before, in front of	premenstrual	period before menstruation
pro-	before, in front of	prophase	first stage of cell division
pros-	before, forward	prosthesis	artificial limb added to the body
post-	after, behind	postmortem	after death

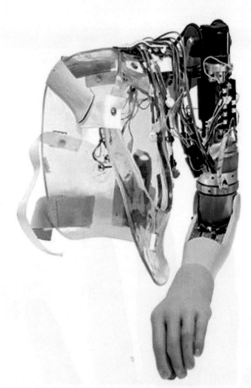

FIGURE 3.4 Prosthesis: a device added to the upper limb after amputation.

It is worth noting that certain prefixes have two meanings. For example, the prefix *ante-* may refer to time and position as in *antepartum* (time) and *antecubital* (position). Similarly, *pro-* refers to time as in *prophase* and position as in *prognathic*. This explains why we place prefixes for time and position together in one list. This will also be noticed in some of the following tables.

Practice 3.4 Define the following terms.

1. projectile _____
2. antefebrile _____
3. postmenopause _____
4. premature _____

Table 3.5 Prefixes for Disease

Prefix	Meaning	Example	Meaning
brady-	slow	bradygastria	decreased rate of electrical pace-maker activity in the stomach
tachy-	fast	tachycardia	rapid heart rhythm
pachy-	thick	pachydactyly	abnormal thickness of the fingers
mal-	bad, poor	malignant	cancerous tumor that spreads like fire
dys-	abnormal, difficult painful, bad/poor	dysplasia, dyspnea dysuria dystrophy	-abnormal development in numbers -difficulty in breathing - painful sensation upon urination - poor development
xero-	dry	xeroma	excessive dryness of the cornea and conjunctiva

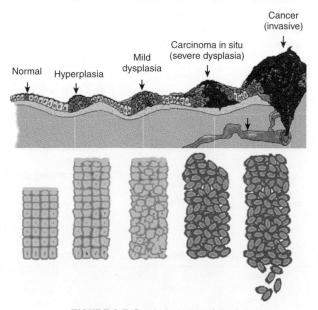

FIGURE 3.5 Dysplasia: stages of dysplasia.

Practice 3.5 The prefix *tachy-* means rapid. Use this prefix in a word that means each of the following:

1. rapid heart rate _____
2. rapid breathing _____
3. extreme rapidity of speech _____
4. abnormally rapid mental activity _____

Table 3.6 Prefixes for Infectious Diseases

Prefix	Meaning	Example	Meaning
staphyl/o-	grapelike cluster	*staphylococcus*	round bacteria that form clusters
strept/o-	twisted chain	*streptobacillus*	a rod-shaped bacterium that forms chains

Table 3.7 Prefixes for Position and Direction

Prefix	Meaning	Example	Meaning
circum-	around	circumcision	circular cut
peri-	around	peritoneal	peritoneum
intra-	within	intravenous	within the vein
extra-	outside	extrahepatic	outside the liver
epi-	above	epidermis	above the skin
supra-	above	supra-abdominal	above the abdomen
infra-	below	infrascapular	below the shoulder blades
sub-	below	subpatellar	below the kneecap
juxta-	near	juxtaposition	a location near another structure
para-	near	parathyroid gland	near the thyroid glands
inter-	between	interstitial	relating to or situated in the small, narrow spaces between tissues or parts of an organ
retro-	behind	retrogastric	behind the stomach

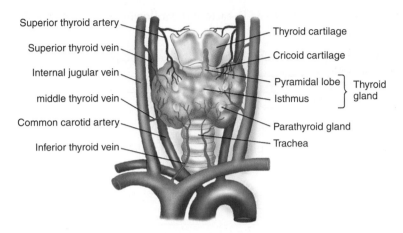

FIGURE 3.6 Parathyroid glands. Four endocrine glands on the posterior of the thyroid gland.

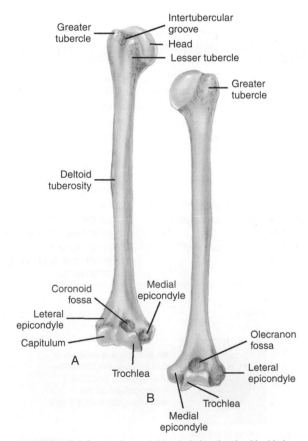

FIGURE 3.7 Infrascapular: pertaining to below the shoulder blades.

Practice 3.6 Replace the prefix in each of the following terms with another one having the same meaning.

1. circumoral _____
2. subcostal _____
3. periorbital _____
4. infrascapular _____

Practice 3.7 Write a word that means the opposite of each of the following terms.

1. suprapatellar _____
2. intracellular _____
3. suprascapular _____
4. hypogastric _____

Table 3.8 Prefixes for Position and Direction

Prefix	Meaning	Example	Meaning
in-, im-	not	insignificant	having no importance
		impermeable	not allowing fluid to pass through
un-	not	unconscious	not aware of one's surroundings
non-	not	nonhuman	not appropriate to human beings
a-, an-	not, lack, without	apnea anemia	cessation of breathing, no blood
anti-	against	antigen	a substance that when introduced into the body stimulates the production of an antibody
contra-	against	contraindicated	against recommendation
de-	down, without, removal	decongestant	a medication or treatment that decreases congestion, as of the sinuses
dis-	removal, separation	disinfect	to cleanse so as to destroy or prevent the growth of disease-carrying microorganisms

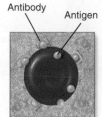

Antibody

Antigen

An antigen is a substance that induces the formation of antibodies because it is recognized by the immune system as a threat

Red blood cell

FIGURE 3.8 Antigen: a foreign substance such as a bacterium or virus.

Practice 3.8 Add a prefix to form the negative of the following words.

1. contributory _____
2. coordinated _____
3. calcify _____
4. compatible _____
5. dote _____
6. sect _____
7. ception _____
8. hydrous _____
9. mnesia_____
10. moral _____

Table 3.9 Prefixes for Position

Prefix	Meaning	Example	Meaning
ecto-	outside	ectocardia	outside the heart
ex/o-	outside	exophthalmos	(Graves disease) protrusion of the eyeball to the outside
dextr/o-	right	dextrogastria	displacement of the stomach to the right
sinister/o-	left	sinistromanual	left handed
end/o-	inside	endometrial	within the uterus
mes/o-	middle	mesoderm	middle layer of a developing embryo
tel/o-	end	telophase	last stage of cell division
tel/e		telencephalon	endbrain
syn-, sym- con-	together	syndrome	- group of signs and symptoms that occur together
		symbiosis	- two dissimilar organisms living together
		congenital	- irregularity present at birth

Table 3.10 Differences between Endocrine and Exocrine Glands

Exocrine Glands	Endocrine Glands
These are enzyme-secreting glands	These are hormone-secreting glands
The activity of the enzymes is short term	The action of released hormones is prolonged
The secreted substances are directly released over the target site or tissue	The secretions are released into blood stream
Some of the examples include sweat glands and gastric glands	Some examples include adrenal gland, pituitary gland and thyroid gland

The major glands that make up the human endocrine system include the:

- hypothalamus
- pituitary gland
- thyroid
- parathyroid
- adrenal glands
- pineal body
- reproductive glands (which include the ovaries and testes)
- pancreas

Examples of exocrine glands:

- salivary glands that secrete saliva into the mouth
- bile-producing glands of the liver
- prostate gland
- the portion of the pancreas that secretes pancreatic fluid into the duodenum
- gastric glands
- sweat glands

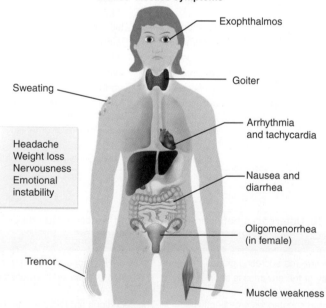

FIGURE 3.9 Exophthaloms: bulging of the eyes.

Practice 3.9 Define the following words.

1. endotoxin _____
2. exogenous _____
3. sympathetic _____
4. synapse _____

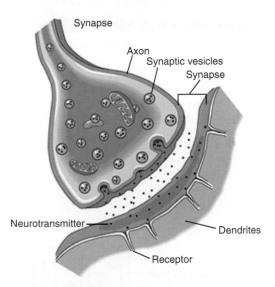

FIGURE 3.10 Synapse: junction between two nerve cells.

Table 3.11 Prefixes for Degree

Prefix	Meaning	Example	Meaning
oligo-	few	oligodontia	less than the normal number of teeth
pan-	all	panplegia	total paralysis
super-	above	supernumerary	in excess number
	excess	superscript	something written above
hyper-	abnormally high	hypertension	high blood pressure
hypo-	abnormally low	hypoglycemia	low blood sugar

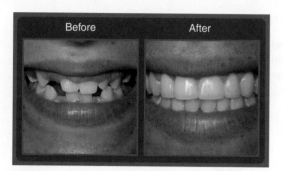

FIGURE 3.11 Oligodontia: having less than the normal number of teeth.

Practice 3.10 The prefix *hyper-* means excessive. Use this prefix to produce a word that means each of the following:

1. overproduction of a hormone _____
2. abnormally deep respiration _____
3. high increase of cells in size _____
4. high increase of cells in numbers _____

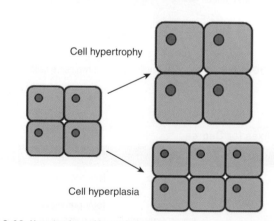

Cell hypertrophy

Cell hyperplasia

FIGURE 3.12 Hypertrophy and hyperplasia: cells increase in size and increase in number.

Table 3.12 Prefixes for Size and Comparison

Prefix	Meaning	Example	Meaning
equi-	equal, same	equicaloric	equal in terms of calories
iso-	equal, same	isochromatic	having the same color
homo- homeo-	same, unchanging	homosexual	- having a sexual orientation to persons of the same sex
		homeostasis	- a property of cells, tissues, and organisms that allows the maintenance and regulation of the stability
hetero-	different, unequal	heterosexual	a person whose sexual orientation is toward people of the opposite sex
macro-	abnormally large	macrodactyly	a condition of abnormally large fingers or toes
mega-, megalo-	abnormally large	megacephaly	- the condition of having an unusually large head or cranial capacity
		megalomania	- a psychopathological condition characterized by delusional fantasies of wealth, power, or omnipotence
micro-	small	microbiological	the branch of biology that deals with microorganisms
eu-	true, good, easy	eupnea	normal breathing
normo-	normal	normothermic	having normal body temperature
ortho-	straight, correct	orthognathism	the condition of having straight jaws
poikilo-	irregular	poikilothermic	having different body temperature
pseudo-	false	pseudogene	a segment of DNA that resembles a gene but is not functional and usually not transcribed
re-	again, back	resection	cutting back and forth in a sense of removal
neo-	new	neocortex	the dorsal region of the cerebral cortex, especially large in primates, thought to have evolved more recently than other parts of the brain

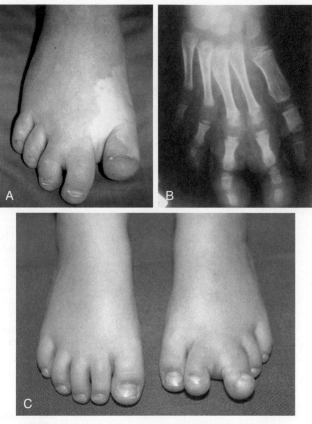

FIGURE 3.13 Macrodactyly: abnormally large fingers or toes.

Practice 3.11 Match each of the following terms in column A with its definition in column B.

A	B
1. isocellular _____	a. composed of different materials
2. homograft _____	b. composed of identical cells
3. normovolemia _____	c. false response
4. heterogeneous _____	d. correcting deformity
5. equilibrium _____	e. return of partly digested food from the stomach to the mouth/backward flow
6. pseudoreaction _____	f. a state of balance

A	B
7. euthyroidism _____	g. normal production of thyroid hormone
8. regurgitation _____	h. large enough to be seen without a microscope
9. poikiloderma _____	i. tissue transplanted to another of the same species
10. macroscopic _____	j. normal blood volume
11. orthotic _____	k. irregular condition of the skin

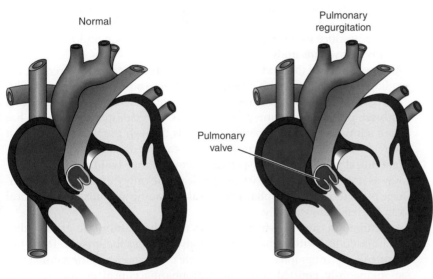

Normal

Pulmonary regurgitation

Pulmonary valve

FIGURE 3.14 Regurgitation: to cause to pour back.

Table 3.13 Terms using different prefixes with the combining forms for fingers (Dactyl/O)

Medical Term	Meaning
syndactyly	a congenital anomaly in humans marked by webbing or fusion of the fingers or toes
polydactyly	a person or animal with digits more than the normal number of digits
oligodactyly	congenital condition in which some fingers or toes are missing
tetradactyly	having four digits on each extremity
monodactyly	an animal with only one digit on each extremity
pachydactyly	enlargement of the fingers or toes, especially extremities
microdactyly	a condition of abnormal smallness of fingers or toes

FOCUS ON READING

Read the following text and answer the questions following it.

Nuclear Concepts Used in Medicine

1. Our bodies are made up of cells in which chemical processes of one form or another constantly occur. Whenever we suffer from an injury or a disease, the affected part of our body cannot properly carry out its chemical functions. In such instances, the diagnostician can introduce a radioactively labeled chemical called a radiopharmaceutical into the affected area, where it will take part in certain of these chemical activities. By detecting the gamma emissions from the radiopharmaceutical employed, we are able to produce useful information about the function and health of the organs that we are studying.

2. Although most of the studies done in clinical nuclear medicine require the radiopharmaceutical to be injected into a vein (normally in the antecubital region), it may on occasion be inhaled, ingested, or injected through a catheter or other implanted device. Once the radiopharmaceutical has been administered to the patient, it travels through the body as though it were normally present. Since our bodies cannot distinguish a radiopharmaceutical from a normally present chemical, they handle it in the same way as it would a nonradioactive chemical. The only difference and advantage offered by the radiopharmaceutical is that the administered chemical can be detected externally.

3. A scintillation camera, which is able to map the distribution of the radiopharmaceutical within the patient's body, provides the images. These images, called scintigraphs or scintiscans, are produced when the gamma rays spontaneously emitted from the radiopharmaceutical escape from the patient's body. Each scintiscan is made up of hundreds of thousands of individual gamma ray interactions with the camera, and these many interactions are displayed as individual dots of light which are added together to form a single image.

4. Typically, images are recorded every 2 s immediately following the injection of the radiopharmaceutical. These initial images provide information about the arterial supply, capillary transit, and venous drainage of the organ or tissue of interest. After a period of time sufficient to permit the tissues to extract the radiopharmaceutical from the circulation, more images are recorded. These first images are called dynamic images, and the latter ones are called statics or delayed images.

5. The radiopharmaceutical used in the study of a particular organ must be chosen for its ability to accumulate in that particular organ. The choice

also depends on the isolation of a chemical pathway or function that is peculiar to the organ that is to **be imaged**. For the most part, the label (the radioactive part of the pharmaceutical) used as a tag within the pharmaceutical does not affect its localization, and so materials are often labeled with gamma emitters that have the best combination of availability, energy, and half-life. A radionuclide called technetium-99m is frequently used because it can be produced onsite from a system called a generator.

6. The process of generation of technetium-99m is a simple one: molybdenum-99 (99Mo) decays to form technetium-99m. Since technetium-99m is chemically different from molybdenum, it is easy to separate the two. A small amount of molybdenum can produce enough technetium each day to meet the needs of a typical nuclear medicine department. Also, technetium-99m emits gamma radiation at an acceptable energy level of 140 KeV. Although this level is higher than most X-rays, human tissue can **tolerate** *it* since gamma rays escape the body, whereas X-rays tend to irradiate body tissues. The final reason for the popularity of this radionuclide is that it has a 6-h half-life long enough to allow the radiopharmaceuticals to accumulate in the tissues of interest and short enough to permit repeat studies within a day or so. The combination of the low energy (by gamma ray standards) and short half-life also gives the patient an acceptably low radiation dose.

7. The radioactivity principle can also be used to detect and measure substances in blood or urine, substances that may be present in such small concentrations that conventional methods cannot detect them. This technique, termed radioimmunoassay (RIA), involves the production of antibodies specific to the substance being measured, the isolation of a pure extract of this substance (termed the antigen), and the radioactive labeling of the antigen. By mixing known amounts of these substances with the patient sample and allowing the whole to come to equilibrium in a test tube, one can separate the unreacted antigen (both from the patient and the labeled antigen) from that which has bound to the antibody provided for that purpose. The ratio of free-to-bound antigens permits a calculation of the amount of material present in the patient's original sample. Tests performed on blood or urine samples requiring that the radioactive chemical be added to the sample but not to the patient are termed **in vitro** tests. Those procedures requiring a radioactive chemical to be administered to the patient are called **in vivo** tests. **In vitro** techniques are commonly used to measure various hormone levels, drug levels, and concentrations of other compounds of medical interest.

A. Answer the following questions:
1. What does the italicized pronoun "it" in **paragraph 6** refer to?
   _____

2. What do the rays emitted from the radiopharmaceutical enable us to do?
   _____

3. What is the main difference between the radiopharmaceutical and the normal chemical in the body?
   _____

4. Define delayed images or "statics."
   _____

5. Summarize **paragraph 5** in one sentence.
   _____

6. What is the difference between **in vitro** tests and **in vivo** tests?
   _____

7. Scan the text and find prefixes that mean
   a. against: _____
   b. before: _____
   c. between: _____
   d. complete: _____

8. Circle the word that is closest in meaning to the highlighted word in **paragraph 6**.

   a. reject   b. accept   c. accumulate   d. radiate

9. Find a word that means "expose to radiation" in **paragraph 6**.
10. What is the meaning of the bold-faced word in **paragraph 5**?

B. Find words in the text that mean:
1. A noun meaning "a person who determines the cause of a disease." (Para. 1)
   _____

2. An adjective meaning "a radioactive compound used in diagnosis or therapy." (Para. 1)
   _____

3. A verb meaning "to take into the body by the mouth for absorption." (Para. 2)
   _____

4. A noun meaning "movement in a circle or circuit, especially the movement of blood through bodily vessels as a result of the heart's pumping action." (Para. 4)
   _____

5. An adjective meaning "not ordinary or usual; odd or strange." (Para. 5)
   _____

6. A verb meaning "to gather or cause to increase." (Para. 6)

_____

7. A noun meaning "the condition existing when a chemical reaction and its reverse reaction proceed at equal rates." (Para. 7)

_____

VOCABULARY DEVELOPMENT

Medical Collocations

Practice 3.12 Match the word in column A with its complement in column B. Write the letter of the correct answer on the line provided.

A	B
1. inoperable _____	a. habits
2. tender _____	b. genes
3. subjective _____	c. tumor
4. premature _____	d. pain
5. genetic _____	e. neck
6. hygienic _____	f. voice
7. hoarse _____	g. report
8. stiff _____	h. infant
9. intermittent _____	i. skin
10. defective _____	j. trait

Practice 3.13 Complete the following sentences using collocations from Practice 3.12.

a. She suffered from _____ after exposing herself to the sun.
b. The doctor provided a _____ on the patient history of his brain tumor.
c. He felt an _____ that kept recurring over and over again.
d. The _____ died due to early birth.
e. The young man dies because of an _____.
f. All doctors have _____ like using disposable tissues.
g. The flu left him with a _____.
h. He awoke with a painful _____.
i. Fixing _____ should be welcome news to those who carry them.
j. The father had a _____ that predisposed him to the development of cancer.

Practice 3.14 Match the words in column A with their collocates in column B. Write the correct answer on the line provided.

A	B
1. enhance _____	a. the onset
2. maintain _____	b. a drug
3. ease _____	c. anxiety
4. identify _____	d. physical fitness
5. induce_____	e. the appetite
6. go into _____	f. infections
7. eradicate _____	g. vomiting
8. tolerate _____	h. antibodies
9. speed _____	i. nausea
10. relieve _____	j. shock

Practice 3.15 What can the following words collocate with?

1. trigger _____
2. enhance _____
3. cleanse _____
4. tolerate _____
5. strain _____

Academic Words

Study the following academic lists.

Academic List 1:

	Words	Definitions
1.	alternative	a choice or course of action that is mutually exclusive with another
2.	philosophy	the attitude or set of ideas that guides the behavior of a person or organization
3.	justify	to give an acceptable explanation for something that other people think is unreasonable
4.	publish	to make official information such as a report available for everyone to read
5.	fund	an amount of money that is collected and kept for a particular purpose
6.	react	to behave in a particular way or show a particular emotion because of something that has happened or been said
7.	techniques	nonprescriptive ways or methods used to perform missions, functions, or tasks
8.	minor	small and not very important or serious, especially when compared with other things
9.	outcome	the final result of a meeting, discussion, etc., used especially when no one knows what it will be until it actually happens
10.	sequence	the order that something happens or exists in, or the order it is supposed to happen or exist in

Academic List 2:

	Words	Definitions
1.	emphasize	to stress, single out as important
2.	coordinate	to organize an activity so that the people involved in it work well together and achieve a good result
3.	ensure	to make certain that something will happen properly
4.	physical	related to someone's body rather than their mind or emotions
5.	compensate	to pay someone money because they have suffered injury, loss, or damage
6.	link	to make a connection between two or more things or people
7.	sufficient	as much as is needed for a particular purpose
8.	criteria	a standard that you use to judge something or make a decision about something
9.	demonstrate	to show or prove something clearly
10.	contribute	to give money, help, ideas, etc. to something that a lot of other people are also involved in

Practice 3.16 Match the words in column A with their definitions in column.

A	B
1. link _____	a. to give an acceptable explanation for something that other people think is unreasonable
2. criterion _____	b. the attitude or set of ideas that guides the behavior of a person or organization
3. publish _____	c. to stress, single out as important
4. justify _____	d. a standard that you use to judge something or make a deci-sion about something
5. philosophy _____	e. the order that something happens or exists in, or the order it is supposed to happen or exist in
6. techniques _____	f. to make a connection between two or more things or people
7. outcome _____	g. to make official information such as a report available for everyone to read
8. emphasize _____	h. to organize an activity so that the people involved in it work well together and achieve a good result
9. sequence _____	i. Nonprescriptive ways or methods used to perform missions, functions, or tasks
10. coordinate _____	j. the final result of a meeting, discussion, etc., used especially when no one knows what it will be until it actually happens

Practice 3.17 Complete each of the following sentences using the correct word from the box.

funded	outcomes	sequential	philosophical	justified
alternative	published	react	techniques	minor

1. His injuries were relatively _____, so he was released from the hospital within a couple of hours of being admitted.
2. Faced with worsening health, and a doctor who did not seem to be able to help him, Ali decided to try _____ medicine.
3. Before we had a publicly _____ universal health care system in Canada, many people could not afford medical care, or faced bankruptcy with a serious illness.
4. Operations on animals helped to develop organ transplant and open-heart surgery _____.
5. Studies have shown that babies in the womb will _____ to sudden loud noises or bright lights that are flashed on the mother's belly.
6. Medical doctors usually take credit for actions which produce favorable _____, but blame the situation when their actions are questionable or lead to failure.
7. My grandfather is very _____ about his illness; he certainly does not want to die, but he says he has lived a long life, and is not afraid to go.
8. We feel that animal testing should be reduced to a minimum and carefully _____ in each case.
9. Protein synthesis is a _____ process in which DNA is transformed into protein.
10. She has _____ a number of important papers in a leading medical journal.

Practice 3.18 Complete each of the following sentences using the correct word from the box.

criteria	compensation	coordinate	demonstrated	emphasize
contributes	physical	sufficiently	ensure	link

1. He _____ a lot of time and money to helping people with Parkinson disease.
2. Students in our medical program will be graded according to the _____ described in the course outline.
3. Eating plenty of fruits, vegetables, protein, and dairy products will _____ your body gets the minerals it needs.
4. He received almost half a million dollars in _____ after his surgical malfunction.
5. Detectives were able to _____ the murderer to the crime using DNA evidence.
6. The Red Cross is trying to _____ relief efforts aimed at aiding the victims of Sunday's earthquake.

7. The best way to lose weight is to do regular _____ activity.
8. Recent studies have _____ that drinking green tea may help to prevent breast cancer.
9. Forgetting material which is stored in long-term memory cannot be _____ explained by the simple passage of time.
10. Doctors usually _____ the need for regular exercise to maintain good health.

FOCUS ON GRAMMAR

Asking Questions

Health care students and practitioners always need to extend their repertoire of medical terminology in order to avoid communication breakdowns with others. They also need more focus on certain grammatical issues such as asking and answering questions and comparing and contrasting drugs and their effects on human body. In this section, students will be reminded of how to ask questions of different types about several medical issues.

Practice 3.19 Study the following questions and learn how to use each highlighted question word. Decide what it is used for and when we can use it.

Who is that man?
Who is the patient?
Who is his next of kin (closest relative)?

When did you hurt your arm?
When do you take your pills?
When did the pain start?

What do you do for a living?
What did you eat yesterday?
What did you do to your leg?
What makes the pain better?
What is the pain like?

How are you?
How are you feeling?
How did you cut yourself?
How strong is the pain?

How long have you been suffering from fever?
How long have you had the pain?

How many tablets do you take a day?
How many cigarettes do you smoke?
How much sleep do you get?

How often do you get regular exercise?
How often do you eat vegetables?

Why did not you follow your doctor's instructions?
Whose medication is this?
Where do you live? **Where** does it hurt you the most?

Practice 3.20 Use each of the above-highlighted question words or phrases in a question of your own on health care issues.

Practice 3.21 Ask questions to which the bold-faced words are answers.

1. The top of a person's **scalp** is covered with **hair**. (What)
   _____

2. At the top and front of the upper body, just below the neck is the **collar bone**. (Where)
   _____

3. The patient takes the medication **three times a day**. (How often)
   _____

4. Jane has been pregnant **for 5 months**. (How long)
   _____

5. The front of the lower leg is the shin and the back of the lower leg is the **calf**. (What)
   _____

6. In many cases **specialists** require a **referral** from a family doctor before they will see a patient. (Who), (What)
   _____
   _____

7. The newborn baby sleeps **four times** every day. (How often)
   _____

8. **Tylenol 3** is one of the painkillers available without prescription. (Which)
   _____

9. **Women giving birth** usually find that the epidural is the most effective pain relief. (Who)
   _____

10. He looks **much worse** today because **the medicines he is taking do not seem to work**. (How), (Why)
    _____
    _____

ORAL COMMUNICATION SKILLS

Practice 3.22 Study the following dialogue between a doctor and a patient and answer the questions following it orally.

Doctor: Hi Janet. How are you feeling today?

Patient: A bit better.

Doctor: That's good to hear. Are you still feeling nauseous?

Patient: No, I haven't felt sick since you switched my medication. My stomach is fine.

Doctor: Great. Say, your test results came in this morning.

Patient: It's about time. Is it good news or bad?

Doctor: I guess it's a bit of both. Which one do you want first?

Patient: Let's get the bad news over with.

Doctor: Okay. It looks like you're going to need surgery to remove the tumor from your leg. After the operation, you're going to have to stay off your feet for at least 3 weeks. That means no soccer.

Patient: I was afraid you were going to say that.

Doctor: Now for the good news. The biopsy shows that the tumor is benign, which means it's not cancerous. We're going to take it out anyway just to be on the safe side.

Patient: Wow, that's a load off my mind. Thanks doctor.

Doctor: Don't get too excited. We still need to get to the bottom of all of this weight loss.

Patient: I've probably just been so worried about this stupid lump.

Doctor: These things often are stress related, but we're still going to do a few blood tests just to rule a few things out.

Patient: Things like what? Cancer?

Doctor: Actually, I'm thinking more along the lines of a food allergy.

A. Answer the following questions.
1. What was the woman suffering from?
2. Why did she have to switch medication?
3. What bad news did the doctor tell her?
4. What medical procedure has the woman already undergone?
5. Define the term *biopsy*.
6. Give the opposite of:
   - *benign:*_____
   - *to lose weight:*_____
B. Act out the dialogue with a classmate.

FOCUS ON WRITING

Definition

Definitions may be brief or extended. A brief definition reflects the essence or primary characteristic of a term. The essence of an adjective, for instance, is that it is a part of speech that modifies a noun. On the other hand, an extended definition includes information beyond the essence or primary characteristic of a term. An extended definition of an adjective could include categories like size, shape, or color, and an explanation of the various forms it takes such as comparative and superlative.

An extended definition essay should classify a term with relevant criteria, and use examples that focus on distinguishing the term from other closely related terms or concepts. The writer must decide what categories of information best distinguish the item or concept under scrutiny.

An appropriate range of examples can be the most direct way to identify and clarify a term.

Example

Alternative medicine incorporates a wide range of substances and systems which include herbal preparations, megadose vitamins, homeopathy, naturopathy, osteopathy, aromatherapy, electromagnetic fields, acupuncture, chiropractic, hypnosis, biofeedback, spiritual devotions, therapeutic touch, chelation therapy, and many more.

This extra information may include the properties of the defined item, an analysis of its parts, a physical description or its location. Furthermore, extra information may focus on the mode of operation of the item to be defined as in defining a diagnostic instrument: *sonography* operates by the energy from sound waves being reflected off internal organs and transformed into an image on a TV-type monitor.

An object can also be clarified by indicating its functions or what is it particularly useful for, or by comparing and contrasting it to other members of the class:

The lung disease "emphysema," which limits a patient's ability to breathe, could be contrasted with "pneumoconiosis," a disease which also results in breathing difficulty, but due to different causes and through a different process.

A definition may also include the causes of the defined item, or its results, or both:

Atherosclerosis is the condition where fatty deposits, called plaque, within the lining of an artery gradually build up and harden, causing a narrowing of the vessel, thereby reducing the blood flow to tissues.

(Result) A primary factor in its development is the presence of cholesterol-containing lipoproteins. Other risk factors include high blood pressure, smoking, inactivity, and family history. (Causes)

Defining a term may involve a description of its process or procedures:

Angioplasty is the procedure commonly used in cases of atherosclerosis. This involves surgically removing the plaque to reopen a narrowed vessel and restore blood flow. The vessel is then kept open by the installation of a stent. This hinged metal or plastic device is inserted into the vessel with a deflated balloon inside it. Once in place, the balloon is inflated and the stent is forced open to a size which will keep the vessel wide. The balloon can then be deflated and removed, whereas the stent remains open and in place.

A medical term can also be defined by stating what it is not:

Alternative medicine incorporates a very broad category of medical systems. However, though it is sometimes treated as synonymous with complementary medicine, they are not the same. Complementary medicine intends to be used as a supplement to conventional treatment. This could involve having vitamin supplements or a health food diet while undergoing conventional medical treatment. On the other hand, alternative systems or treatments function to replace a conventional treatment. Acupuncture could be used instead of anesthesia during an operation. In some countries, like the USA and Britain, alternative medicine is not taught in medical schools, is generally not used in hospitals, and is not covered by insurance. Many conventional medical professionals reject their safety and efficacy. Despite this, there is some professional interest. There are surgeons in the countries mentioned who use acupuncture instead of anesthesia, for instance, in the UAE, there is a government department which deals with alternative medicine. It is fair to say that its status is not fixed.

Practice 3.23 Write an extended definition of one of the following:

a. Endocrine glands
b. Exocrine glands
c. Graves disease
d. Colonoscopy

PRONUNCIATION OF MEDICAL TERMS

The following are the medical terms introduced in this chapter. You are supposed to read them aloud as many times as you need to master their pronunciations. In this activity, you are also required to give the meaning of each term in order to retain them active in your memory.

Read the following medical terms and know their meanings.

abduct	eupnea
adduct	euthyroidism
adhere	exogenous
adjacent	exophthalmos
amenorrhea	extracranial
anemia	extrahepatic
antefebrile	hemiplegia
antepartum	heterogeneous
antigen	heterosexual
aphasia	homeostasis
apnea	homograft
atrophy	homosexual
bilateral	hypertension
bipolar	hyperthyroidism
bradygastria	hypochondriac
circumcision	hypogastric
circumoral	hypoglycemia
congenital	hypothyroidism
contraindicated	incision
cyanosis	infrascapular
decongestant	interstitial
dextrogastria	intervertebral
dialysis	intracellular
diameter	intrauterine
diatomic	intravenous
diploid	isocellular
diplopic	isochromatic
disinfect	juxtaposition
dysplasia	leukemia
dyspnea	leukoplakia
dysuria	macrodactyly
ectocardia	macroscopic
ectopic	malignant
endocrine	megacephaly
endometrial	megalomania
endotoxin	melanin
epidermis	melanocyte
equicaloric	mesoderm
equilibrium	metacarpal
erythrocyte	microbiological
erythrocytosis	microdactyly

monoatomic
monocular
monodactyly
multicellular
neocortex
nonhuman
normothermic
normovolemia
oligodactyly
oligodontia
orthognathism
orthotic
pachydactyly
panplegia
parathyroid gland
percolate
perianal
periorbital
peritoneal
permeable
poikiloderma Graves disease

poikilothermic
poliomyelitis
polydactyly
polyneuropathy polyphagia
postmenopause
postmortem
postnatal
tachycardia
telencephalon
telophase
tetrad
tetradactyly
transdermal
transurethral
tripod
ultrasonography
unilateral
xanthoderma
xanthoma
xeroma

REVIEW EXERCISES

A. **Circle the best answer.**

1. A prefix that means the same as *di-* is
   a. tri   b. uni   c. bi   d. mono
2. The prefixes *hemi-* and *semi-* mean
   a. whole   b. first   c. two   d. half
3. The prefix in *binocular* means
   a. one   b. three   c. four   d. two
4. The prefix in *nonexistent* means
   a. slow   b. complex   c. equal   d. not
5. A *neonate* is a/an
   a. teen   b. adult   c. preteen   d. newborn
6. The prefixes *ante-*, *pre-*, and *pro-* all mean
   a. after   b. within   c. under   d. before
7. The prefix *tel/o-* means
   a. together   b. middle   c. end   d. apart
8. The prefixes *meta-* and *ultra-* mean
   a. whole   b. outside   c. inside   d. beyond

9. The prefix in *analysis* means
   a. apart   b. not   c. separation   d. breaking
10. The prefix in *pachycephaly* means
   a. slow   b. fast   c. equal   d. thickness

B. Write true or false before each statement.

1. _____ The prefix in *leukocyte* means "irregular."
2. _____ The prefix in *percutaneous* means "on the skin."
3. _____ The prefix in *synthesis* means "apart."
4. _____ The last stage of cell division is prophase.
5. _____ A prefix appears before a root and after a suffix.
6. _____ A polysaccharide is composed of more sugar than a monosaccharide.
7. _____ The prefix in *dissect* means "to separate."
8. _____ "Anti-" and "contra-" mean the same thing.
9. _____ Right-handed people are dextromanual.
10. _____ A telomere is found in the middle of a chromosome.
11. _____ The prefix in *erythrocyte* means "red."
12. _____ The prefix in *periosteum* means "on the bone."

C. Fill in the blank with the correct medical term.

1. Hypoxia causes a bluish discoloration of the skin termed _____.
2. The prefix in *superciliary* means _____.
3. The prefix *poikilo-* means _____.
4. The prefix in the word *pachycephaly* means _____.
5. Total paralysis _____.
6. Composed of similar cells _____.
7. A group of four _____.
8. Describing a colony derived from one cell _____.
9. To separate tissues for anatomical study _____.
10. A mass of blood above the membrane surrounding the brain is _____.
11. Surgical puncture to remove fluid from the membrane surrounding the fetus is _____.

D. Write the word that means the opposite of each of the following:

1. hyperthermia _____
2. polyuria _____
3. incision _____
4. abduct _____
5. chronic _____
6. benign _____
7. hypnea _____

  8. acute _____

  9. malignant _____

 10. atrophy _____

 11. bradypnea _____

E. Identify the prefix and provide its meaning.

Prefix	Meaning
1. normothermic _____	_____
2. quadruplet _____	_____
3. mesoderm _____	_____
4. euthyroidism _____	_____
5. poikilothermic _____	_____
6. malabsorption _____	_____
7. symbiosis _____	_____
8. panplegia _____	_____

F. Write a word or a prefix that means the same as each of the following:

1. isolateral _____

2. megalocyte _____

3. supersensitivity _____

4. prenatal _____

5. para- _____

6. circum- _____

7. subcostal _____

8. exo- _____

G. Identify the prefixes or the combining forms in the following words and figure out what they mean.

	Term	Prefix	Combining Form	Meaning
1.	oliguria			
2.	cyanosis			
3.	erythropenia			
4.	leukorrhea			
5.	melanocyte			
6.	endocrine			
7.	fibroid			
8.	morphology			
9.	aphasia			
10.	dysplasia			
11.	eupnea			
12.	peritoneum			
13.	endoscopy			
14.	angioectasis			

H. **Give the meaning of each of the following terms:**
1. sublingual _____
2. retroperitoneal _____
3. aphasia _____
4. quadriplegia _____
5. intervertebral _____
6. hypochondriac _____
7. hypertension _____
8. congenital _____
9. dystrophy _____
10. transdermal _____
11. diplopia _____
12. polyphagia _____
13. postmortem _____
14. tachycardia _____
15. sinistromanual _____

I. **Give the meaning of each of the following prefixes and give a medical term in which it is used.**

Meaning	Example
1. ab- _____	_____
2. ad- _____	_____
3. meta- _____	_____
4. para- _____	_____
5. con- _____	_____
6. anti- _____	_____
7. ante- _____	_____
8. inter- _____	_____
9. brady- _____	_____
10. pre- _____	_____
11. sub- _____	_____
12. hyper- _____	_____
13. dys- _____	_____
14. ec- _____	_____
15. intra- _____	_____
16. syn- _____	_____
17. epi- _____	_____
18. extra- _____	_____
19. trans- _____	_____
20. endo- _____	_____

J. Circle the correct answer.

1. A prefix is found
   a. at the beginning of a word
   b. after the root
   c. at the end of the word
   d. before a hyphen

2. The prefix multi- means
   a. single
   b. double
   c. twice
   c. many

3. Which of the following has four components?
   a. unicycle
   b. polysaccharide
   c. bicuspid
   d. tetralogy

4. Cyanosis refers to
   a. dark coloration
   b. blue coloration
   c. thickness
   d. shape

5. A xanthoma is
   a. green
   b. blue
   c. dark
   d. yellow

6. The prefix in disintegration means
   a. movement
   b. separation
   c. few
   d. decreased

7. To detoxify means to
   a. poison
   b. confine
   c. remove toxins
   d. manufacture toxins

8. The prefixes dia-, per-, and trans- all mean
   a. under
   b. near
   c. through
   d. equal

9. The prefix pan- means
   a. ever
   b. before
   c. excess
   d. all
10. Which of the following means the same as equi-?
   a. pseudo
   b. megalo
   c. ecto
   d. iso
11. The prefix pseudo- means
   a. good
   b. large
   c. even
   d. false
12. The opposite of dextro- is
   a. telo
   b. sym
   c. megalo
   d. sinistro
13. The opposite of ectoderm is
   a. endoderm
   b. proderm
   c. mesoderm
   d. metroderm
14. The mesencephalon is the
   a. surface of the brain
   b. underneath part of the brain
   c. inner part of the brain
   d. middle portion of the brain
15. A word that describes organisms living together is
   a. symbiosis
   b. antibiosis
   c. metabiosis
   d. endobiosis
16. Interstitial fluid is found
   a. inside cells
   b. between cells
   c. on the surface of the skin
   d. under the brain
17. Metastasis is
   a. a wasting of tissue
   b. a form of anemia
   c. a form of infection
   d. spreading of cancer

18. An antipyretic is used to
    a. increase body temperature
    b. harden bones
    c. reduce pain
    d. reduce fever
19. An endotoxin is a
    a. poison found within a cell
    b. spreading cancer cell
    c. substance produced by the immune system
    d. poison secreted from a cell
20. The opposite of bradycardia is
    a. dyscardia
    b. xerocardia
    c. cardiocele
    d. tachycardia
21. In pachyemia, the blood is
    a. thin
    b. light
    c. deficient
    d. thick
22. The term hyperbaric refers to
    a. increased temperature
    b. increased pressure
    c. treatment with chemicals
    d. decreased pressure
23. When a drug is contraindicated, it is
    a. given in double dose
    b. given at night
    c. recommended for treatment
    d. not recommended for treatment
24. Polyarteritis is
    a. constriction of two arteries
    b. inflammation of many arteries
    c. formation of tissue around arteries
    d. removal of tissue from an artery
25. The scientific term for a "heart attack" is
    a. myocardial infarction
    b. endocarditis
    c. pericardial occlusion
    d. cardioversion
26. The epiglottis is the
    a. lower end of the trachea
    b. throat
    c. cartilage around the bronchioles
    d. cartilage that covers the trachea during swallowing

27. Orthopnea is
    a. a rapid rate of breathing
    b. a shallow depth of breathing
    c. irregular breathing
    d. difficulty in breathing unless upright
28. A decreased rate and depth of breathing is termed
    a. hyperpnea
    b. hypocapnia
    c. hyperventilation
    d. hypopnea
29. A temporary stoppage of breathing is
    a. apnea
    b. dyspnea
    c. dysventilation
    d. eupnea
30. The term perioral means
    a. above the nose
    b. within the sinuses
    c. around the mouth
    d. around the jaw
31. The term hemiglossal refers to
    a. the salivary glands in the cheek
    b. the position of the jaw
    c. one-half of the tongue
    d. the upper part of the palate
32. Oliguria is
    a. excretion of a decreased amount of urine
    b. discoloration of the urine
    c. infection of the bladder
    d. narrowing of the ureter
33. Painful or difficult urination is
    a. nocturia
    b. pyuria
    c. uremia
    d. dysuria
34. A retrouterine structure is located
    a. under the uterus
    b. behind the vagina
    c. behind the uterus
    d. within the uterus
35. A congenital disorder
    a. is caused by viral infection
    b. is present at birth
    c. appears during childhood
    d. appears in a mother

K. Case report

Case study: HIV infection and tuberculosis

T.H., a 48-year-old man, was an admitted intravenous (i.v.) drug user and occasionally abused alcohol. Over 4 weeks, he had experienced fever, night sweats, malaise, a cough, and a 10-lb weight loss. He was also concerned about several discolored lesions that had erupted weeks before on his arms and legs.

T.H. made an appointment with a physician assistant (PA) at the neighborhood clinic. On examination, the PA noted bilateral anterior cervical and axillary lymphadenopathy and pyrexia. T.H.'s temperature was 39°C. The PA sent T.H. to the hospital for further studies.

T.H.'s chest radiograph (X-ray image) showed paratracheal adenopathy and bilateral interstitial infiltrates, suspicious of tuberculosis (TB). His blood study results were positive for human immunodeficiency virus (HIV) and showed a low lymphocyte count. Sputum and bronchobacillus (AFB); a PPD (purified protein derivative) skin test result was also positive. On the basis of these findings, T.H. was diagnosed with HIV, TB, and Kaposi sarcoma related to past i.v. drug abuse.

a. **Write the word or phrase from the text that has the same meaning as each of the following words or phrases:**
   1. within a vein _____.
   2. hyperthermia _____.
   3. pertaining to both sides _____.
   4. pertaining to the neck _____.
   5. pertaining to the armpit _____.
   6. X-ray image _____.
   7. near the trachea _____.
   8. backward flow _____.

b. **Circle the letter of the most appropriate answer.**
   1. The term lymphadenopathy means
      a. a disease of the lymph
      b. an enlargement of the lymph nodes, usually associated with disease
      c. lymph nodes enlargement
      d. a disease of a gland
   2. The term interstitial means
      a. above the cells
      b. under the cells
      c. between the cells
      d. within the cells
   3. The word discolored has the prefix
      a. di
      b. dis
      c. ed
      d. color

4. Provide the meaning for the following words:
   a. immunodeficiency _____
   b. infiltrate _____
   c. sarcoma _____
   d. adenopathy _____

SELF-ASSESSMENT

Check (✓) what you learned. If you need more information or practice, refer to the relevant section in the chapter.

( ) I can define a prefix.
( ) I can identify prefixes in medical terms.
( ) I can differentiate between the prefixes that have similar meanings.
( ) I can analyze medical terms into their constituents.
( ) I can use prefixes in medical terms.
( ) I can use certain medical collocations and academic words properly.
( ) I can pronounce medical terms properly.
( ) I can skim and scan medical texts for main ideas and details.
( ) I can ask and answer questions pertaining to medical issues.
( ) I can write brief definitions of medical terms, procedures, disease, etc.
( ) I can spell and pronounce the new medical terms in the chapter.

CHAPTER 4

Body Structure

LEARNING OUTCOMES

By the end of this chapter, students are expected to:

1. name the body systems
2. identify directional terms
3. describe body planes
4. identify body cavities and name the organs within each
5. identify body regions and name the organs within each
6. describe body positions used in medical practice
7. define medical terms pertaining to body structure
8. analyze, pronounce, and spell new medical terms
9. write an extended definition

BODY STRUCTURE

The human body consists of small parts called cells or atoms that assemble together to form larger structures that can be studied at different levels of organization. The levels of organization from least to most complex are cell, tissue, organ, system, and organism. The human body consists of different types of tissue. Histology is the branch of biology that studies the microscopic structure of tissues. There are four main types of tissues in the body: lining cells (epithelia), connective tissue, nervous tissue, and muscle tissue. These tissues finally compose body organs and systems. The study of the human body involves the study of its anatomy, physiology, histology, and embryology. Anatomy is the science dealing with the form and structure of living organisms, whereas physiology is concerned with the systems and organs of the human body and their functions. Histology is study of the minute structure of cells, tissues, and organisms in relation to their function (microscopic anatomy). Finally, embryology is the branch of biology and medicine concerned with the study of embryos and their development.

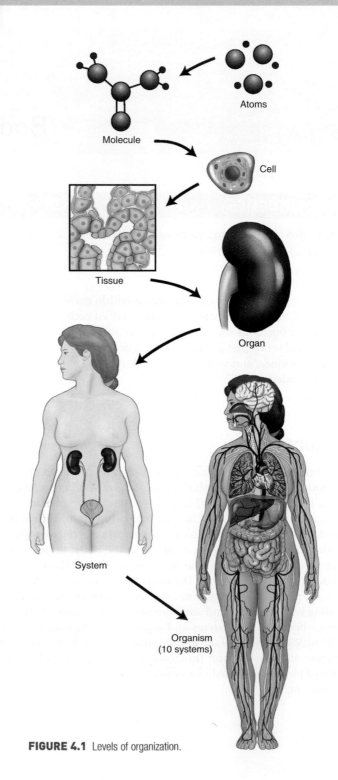

FIGURE 4.1 Levels of organization.

The major components of the human body are the head, the neck, and the trunk which involves the thorax, the abdomen, hands, legs, and feet. For health care students and practitioners, the human body can be studied in terms of anatomical direction or location of a certain point or organ, body planes, cavities, regions, and positions. Knowing the anatomical terms is essential to professionals in all health care careers because they need to know how the human body functions. Furthermore, they are bound to use such terms in order to effectively care for their clients.

Combining Forms

The following is a list of some combining forms related to body structure.

Please note that a few combining forms are repeated from previous chapters as a reminder when you go through this chapter.

Combining Form	Meaning	Example
acr/o	extremity	acrocyanosis
albin/o	white	albinism
anter/o	front	anterior
brachi/o	arm	antebrachium
caud/o	tail	caudal
cephal/o	head	cephalic
cervic/o	neck	cervical
chlor/o	green	chloropia
chondr/o	cartilage	hypochondriac
chrom/o	color	heterochromic
cirrh/o	yellow	cirrhosis
coccyg/o	tailbone	coccygeal
crani/o	skull	craniotomy
dactyl/o	finger, toe	polydactyly
dist/o	far/further	distal
dors/o	back (of body)	dorsal
eti/o	cause	etiology
femor/o	thighbone	femoral
idi/o	unknown	idiopathic
ili/o	flaring portion of hip bone	ilium
infer/o	lower, below	inferior
inguin/o	groin	inguinal
ischi/o	ischium	lower portion of hip bone
jaund/o	yellow	jaundice
lapar/o	abdominal wall	laparoscopy
later/o	side	lateral

Combining Form	Meaning	Example
lumb/o	loins (lower back)	lumbar
medi/o	middle	mediad
mediastin/o	space between the lungs	mediastinum
morph/o	form, shape	polymorphus
pelv/o	pelvis	pelvic
pelvi/o	pelvis	pelvimeter
peritone/o	peritoneum	peritoneal cavity
phren/o	diaphragm	phrenectomy
pleur/o	membrane surrounding the lung	pleurodesis
pod/o	foot	podiatry
poster/o	back (of body)	posterior
proxim/o	near/nearer	proximal
sacr/o	five fused bones in the lower back	sacrum
somat/o	body	somatic
spin/o	spine	spinal
thorac/o	chest	thoracic
trache/o	windpipe	tracheotomy
umbilic/o	navel	umbilical
ventr/o	belly side	ventral
viscer/o	internal organs	visceral
xer/o	dry	xerosis

PRINCIPAL BODY SYSTEMS

A group of organs that work together to perform one of the major functions of the body form a system. There are 11 systems in the body, and each plays an essential role in the way the body works.

1. The **integumentary system** includes the skin and its appendages such as the hair, nails, and sweat and oil glands. It protects the body from various kinds of damage, such as loss of water or abrasion from outside.
2. The **musculoskeletal system** consists of all the bones of the body (206) and their associated cartilages, muscles, tendons, ligaments, and joints. This system provides form, stability, and support to the body. It also enables the body to move.
3. The **cardiovascular system** consists of the heart, blood, and blood vessels. It transports oxygen and nutrients to the body tissues and helps the body to dispose of metabolic wastes. It is also called the circulatory system.
4. The **lymphatic system** works in close cooperation with the circulatory system. It consists of the lymph, lymphatic vessels, and the spleen.

5. The **nervous system** consists of the brain, spinal cord, nerves, and sense organs, such as the eye and ear and all the nerves that connect these organs with the body. It is responsible for the control and communication among its various parts.

6. The **endocrine system** includes all hormone-producing glands and cells such as the pituitary gland, thyroid gland, and pancreas. It regulates body functions by means of hormones.

7. The **respiratory system** includes the nose, pharynx, larynx, trachea, bronchi, and lungs. It transports air in and out of the lungs. It facilitates the diffusion of the oxygen into the blood stream. It also receives carbon dioxide from the blood and exhales it.

8. The **digestive system** starts at the oral cavity including the teeth, the tongue, salivary glands, pharynx, esophagus, stomach, liver, gallbladder and pancreas, small and large intestines, and ends with the anus. This long tract is called the alimentary canal or the gastrointestinal (GI) tract. This system breaks down and absorbs food for use by cells and eliminates solid and other waste.

9. The **urinary system**, also known as the renal system, consists of the kidneys, ureters, bladder, and the urethra. The major function of this system is to remove liquid waste from the blood in the form of urine and to keep a stable balance of salts and other substances in the blood.

10. The **immune system** is made up of a network of cells such as the white blood cells, tissues, and organs that function together in order to protect the body from organisms that may cause diseases.

11. The **reproductive system** of males consists of the testes, prostate glands, sperm ducts, urethra, and penis. The female reproductive system consists of the vagina, uterus, ovaries, and fallopian tubes. Each system has its own functions that serve the general reproduction function in both males and females.

Practice 4.1 Match each of the following body systems in column A with its function in column B.

A	B
1 cardiovascular system _____	a. performs breathing
2 digestive system _____	b. removes fluid and resolves waste
3 endocrine system _____	c. sends and receives messages
4 integumentary system _____	d. pumps and circulates blood to tissues
5 lymphatic and immune system _____	e. covers the body and its internal structures
6 musculoskeletal system _____	f. provides defenses for the body

A	B
7 nervous system _____	g. breaks down food
8 reproductive system _____	h. secretes hormones within the body and into the bloodstream
9 respiratory system _____	i. controls reproduction
10 urinary system _____	j. supports the body and allows it to move

Practice 4.2 Complete the sentences.

1. The system that protects the body from organisms that may cause diseases is the _____.
2. That system that transports blood throughout the body is the _____.
3. The system that brings food into the body and breaks it down is the _____.
4. The system that produces the cells that join to form the embryo is the _____.
5. The system that controls breathing is the _____.
6. The system that produces urine and sends it out of the body is the _____.
7. The system that receives messages from the environment and sends them to the brain is the _____.
8. The system that carries messages to and from the brain is the _____.

PLANES OF THE BODY

This section will present the major body planes and directional terms that allow us to explain the position of one body part compared to another. It is necessary to remember that anatomical positions and directional terms were introduced in order to enable health care providers to describe body parts and positions correctly. The reference point for all these terms and directions is the standard body position that is referred to as the **anatomical position** in which the body is erect (standing straight), facing forward, upper limbs at side and palms facing forward, and the feet parallel.

Body planes are imaginary vertical and horizontal lines that are used to divide the body in the anatomic position into sections for descriptive purposes. Knowing these planes would enable you to read and interpret imaging studies such as MRI, CT scans, and X-rays.

The three planes of the body are as follows:

1. **Frontal or coronal plane** is a vertical plane that runs through the center of your body from side to side. This plane divides the body into front (anterior) and back (posterior) regions.

2. **Lateral or sagittal plane** is a vertical plane that runs through your body from front to back or back to front. This plane divides the body into right and left regions. **Median or midsagittal plane** is a plane that divides the body into **equal** right and left regions. Parasagittal plane is a plane that divides the body into **unequal** right and left regions.
3. **Transverse or axial plane is** a horizontal plane that runs through the midsection of your body. This plane divides the body into upper (superior) and lower (inferior) regions.

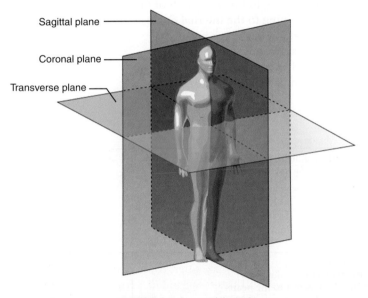

Sagittal plane

Coronal plane

Transverse plane

FIGURE 4.2 Planes of the body.

ORIENTATION AND DIRECTIONAL TERMS

Directional terms are used to show the position of a structure in relation to another structure.

- **Superior (cranial)**: toward the head or upper part of the body; above
- **Inferior (caudal)**: away from the head or toward the lower part of the body; below
- **Ventral (anterior)**: toward or at the front of the body; in front of
- **Dorsal (posterior)**: toward or at the back of the body; behind

- **Medial**: toward or at the midline of the body
- **Lateral**: away from the midline of the body
- **Intermediate**: between a medial and lateral position
- **Proximal**: closer to the origin of the body part or point of attachment of a limb to the body trunk
- **Distal**: away from the origin of a body part or point of attachment of a limb to the body trunk
- **Superficial (external)**: toward or at the body surface
- **Deep (internal)**: away from the body surface
- **Abduction**: movement away from the median plane of the body
- **Adduction**: movement toward the median plane of the body
- **Parietal**: pertaining to the outer wall of the body cavity
- **Visceral**: pertaining to the internal organs
- **Inversion**: turning inward or inside out
- **Eversion**: turning outward
- **Palmar**: pertaining to the palm of the hand
- **Plantar**: pertaining to the sole of the foot

anatomical position	body is standing straight, facing forward, upper limbs at side, and palms facing forward	
anterior (ventral)	toward the front the eyes are anterior to the brain the sternum is anterior to the heart	
posterior	toward the back; opposite of anterior the esophagus is posterior to the trachea	

superior	a body part is above another part, or is closer to the head the heart is superior to the liver	
inferior	a body part is below another body part, is toward the feet the stomach is inferior to the lungs	
medial	closer to midline the ulna is on the medial side of the arm	
lateral	away from midline the arms are lateral to the chest	
proximal	toward origin or trunk the humerus is proximal to the radius	
distal	away from the origin or trunk the phalanges are distal to the carpals	
superficial	toward surface of body the skin is superficial to the skeletal muscle	

Continued

deep	inward from body surface; toward core the lungs are deep to the skin	
intermediate	between a medial and lateral position the collarbone is intermediate between breastbone and shoulder	
bilateral	paired structures, one on each side	
ipsilateral	structures on the same side	*the liver is ipsilateral to the appendix*
contralateral	structures on the opposite side	*the spleen is contralateral to the liver*

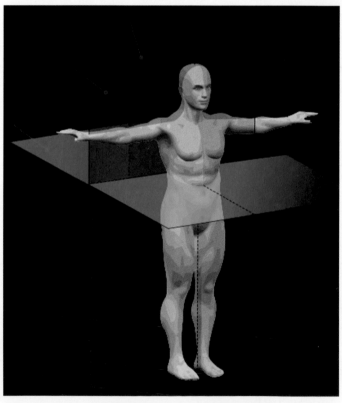

FIGURE 4.3 Directional terms.

Practice 4.3 Look at the following figure and answer the questions following it by circling the letter of the correct answer.

1. Which plane is indicated in RED?

    a. transverse plane   b. frontal plane

    c. sagittal plane   d. axial plane

2. Which plane is indicated in BLUE?

    a. sagittal plane   b. coronary plane

    c. frontal plane   d. transverse plane

3. Which plane is indicated in GREEN?

    a. transverse plane   b. midline plane

    c. sagittal plane   d. medial plane

Practice 4.4 Circle the correct answer.

1. The areas on the front and back of the hand are _____ and _____, respectively.

    a. palmar and dorsal   b. dorsal and palmar

    c. proximal and palmar   d. distal and proximal

2. The areas of the hand which are closer to the body are referred to as _____ and those further away are referred to as _____.

    a. distal and proximal   b. dorsal and proximal

    c. proximal and distal   d. palmar and distal

3. The transverse plane divides the body into _____ and _____ portions.

    a. top and bottom   b. posterior and anterior

    c. proximal and distal   d. superior and inferior

4. The sagittal plane divides the body into _____ and _____. The terms used to describe the distance to this dividing plane are _____ and _____.

    a. back and front; medial and   b. front and back; posterior and
       lateral   anterior

    c. left and right; medial and lateral   d. left and right; posterior and
                                              anterior

5. The coronal plane divides the body into _____ and _____ portions.

    a. left and right   b. posterior and anterior

    c. above and below   d. medial and proximal

6. The terms used to describe areas that are, for instance, close to the surface of the skin or further inside the body are _____ and _____.

    a. superficial and deep   b. inner and outer

    c. anterior and distal   d. proximal and posterior

BODY POSITIONS

They refer to the different physical configurations that the human body can take.

- **Lithotomy position**: in this position, the body is lying in a supine position with hips and knees fully extended. The feet are strapped in position to support the flexed knees and hips.
- **Supine position**: in this position, the body is lying down with face pointing upward. All the remaining positions are similar to anatomical position with the only difference of being in a horizontal plane rather than a vertical plane.
- **Prone position**: this is the position in which the back of the body is directed upward. The body lies in a horizontal plane with face directed downward.
- **Dorsal recumbent:** patient lying on back with knees bent and feet flat on the examination table.
- **Knee-chest:** patient face down with head, chest, and knees on examination table, knees bent with rear end up in the air.
- **Sims' (also known as left lateral) position:** patient lying on left side with left arm behind back, right hip and knee flexed.
- **Trendelenburg:** patient lies in a supine position at an angle with head lower than trunk, and knees bent.
- **Modified Trendelenburg:** patient lies supine at an angle with head lower than trunk, but knees straight.
- **Sitting:** patient sits upright on examination table with knees bent over table edge; feet may be resting on footrest.
- **Fowler's position:** patient sits upright on examination table with legs extended, trunk at a 90-degree angle with back supported. Knees may be elevated.
- **Decubitus position:** lying down, specifically according to the part of the body resting on a flat surface, as in left or right lateral decubitus, or dorsal or ventral decubitus.
- **Left lateral recumbent:** on left side, right leg drawn up.
- **Right lateral recumbent:** the right lateral recumbent, or RLR, means that the patient is lying on their right side.

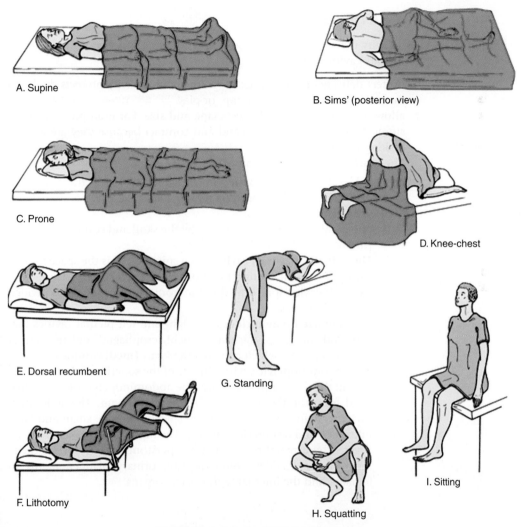

A. Supine

B. Sims' (posterior view)

C. Prone

D. Knee-chest

E. Dorsal recumbent

F. Lithotomy

G. Standing

H. Squatting

I. Sitting

FIGURE 4.4 Illustration of different body positions.

BODY CAVITIES

A body cavity is a space within the body that contains and protects the internal organs. Body cavities can:

a. protect delicate organs. For example, the cranial cavity protects the brain from shocks when we walk, jump, or play.
b. allow internal organs to change shape and size. For example, our lungs, stomach, and bladder can expand and contract because they are located inside cavities.

There are two major cavities in the body:

1. **The dorsal cavity**: it is located in the skull and within the spinal column. The dorsal cavity protects the organs of the nervous system and it includes two subcavities:
   a. **The cranial cavity** is surrounded by the skull and contains the brain (brain case).
   b. **The spinal (vertebral) cavity** or the spinal canal is the space located within the spinal column that houses the spinal cord.
2. **The ventral cavity**: it is located in the front of the body and is divided into two subcavities:
   a. **The thoracic cavity** includes the right and left pleural cavities that surround the lungs, trachea, bronchi, esophagus, and the central pericardial cavity which contains the heart **(mediastinum)**.
   b. **The abdominopelvic cavity** consists of the superior **abdominal** cavity and the inferior **pelvic** cavity. The abdominopelvic cavity is separated from the thoracic cavity by the **diaphragm**. The abdominal cavity contains the stomach, liver, spleen, kidneys, small and large intestines, and ovaries (in females). The organs within this cavity are covered by a membrane called the **peritoneum**. The pelvic cavity includes the bladder, colon, rectum, urinary bladder, uterus in females, and the internal reproductive organs.

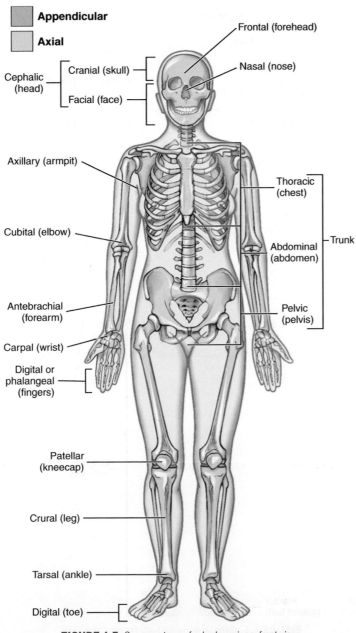

FIGURE 4.5 Common terms for body regions, front view.

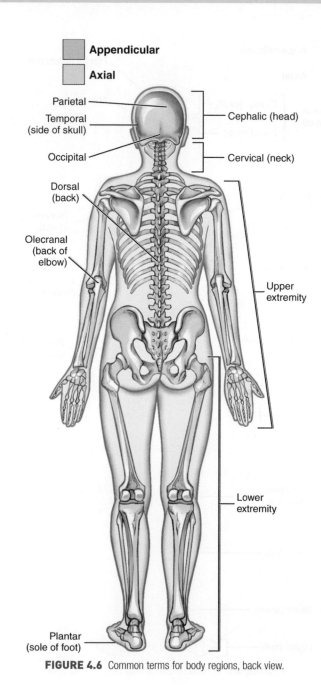

FIGURE 4.6 Common terms for body regions, back view.

Other body cavities include:

1. Oral and digestive: mouth and cavities of the digestive organs
2. Nasal: located within and posterior to the nose
3. Orbital: houses the eyes
4. Middle ear: bones that transmit sound vibration
5. Synovial: joint cavities

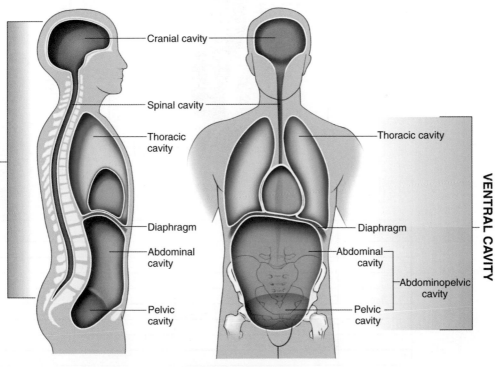

FIGURE 4.7 Body cavities.

Practice 4.5 Label each numbered part. Write its name in the table below.

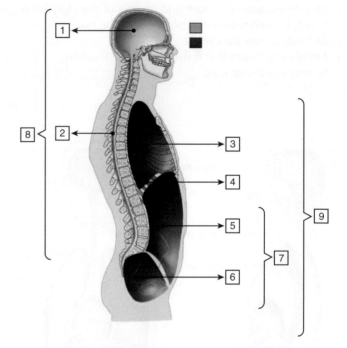

	Name
1	
2	
3	
4	
5	
6	
7	
8	
9	

Abdominal Regions

The abdominal area lies beneath the diaphragm. It holds the organs of digestion and the organs of reproduction and excretion. Two anatomical methods are used to divide this area of the body for medical purposes.

    A. **Regions**. The abdominal regions can be divided by imaginary lines into nine regions: three medial and six lateral.
       The three medial regions are as follows:

        1. **Epigastric:** The epigastric region is above the stomach region. This region pushes out when the diaphragm contracts during breathing.

2. **Umbilical:** The umbilical region contains the umbilicus (navel).
3. **Hypogastric:** The hypogastric region is below the stomach.

The six lateral regions are as follows:

1. **Right hypochondriac:** The right hypochondriac region is the upper right region beneath the ribs.
2. **Left hypochondriac:** The left hypochondriac region is the upper left region beneath the ribs.
3. **Right lumbar:** The right lumbar region is the right middle lateral region.
4. **Left lumbar:** The left lumbar region is the left middle lateral region.
5. **Right iliac (inguinal):** The right iliac region is the right lower lateral region.
6. **Left iliac (inguinal):** The left iliac region is the left lower lateral region.

B. **Quadrants:** Dividing the abdomen into four imaginary quadrants makes it easier to describe where an abdominal organ is located.
   - The **right upper quadrant** or **RUQ** is on the right upper anterior side.
   - The **right lower quadrant** or **RLQ** is on the right lower anterior side.
   - The **left upper quadrant** or **LUQ** is on the left upper anterior side.
   - The **left lower quadrant** or **LLQ** is on the left lower anterior side.

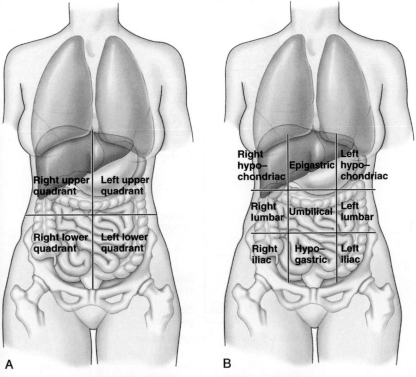

FIGURE 4.8 Abdominopelvic regions and quadrants.

Divisions of the Back

The spinal column is a long row of bones (33 individual bones) from the neck to the tailbone. The vertebrae are numbered and divided into regions: cervical, thoracic, lumbar, sacrum, and coccyx. Only the top 24 bones are moveable; the vertebrae of the sacrum and coccyx are fused. The vertebrae in each region have unique features that help them perform their main functions.

1. **Cervical** (neck): The main function of the cervical spine is to support the weight of the head (C1–C7).
2. **Thoracic** (chest): The main function of the thoracic spine is to hold the rib cage and protect the heart and lungs (T1–T12).
3. **Lumbar** (loin or waist): The main function of the lumbar spine is to bear the weight of the body (L1–L5).
4. **Sacral** (lower back): The main function of the sacrum is to connect the spine to the hip bones (iliac). There are five sacral vertebrae, which are fused together.
5. **Coccygeal** (tailbone): The four fused bones of the coccyx or tailbone provide attachment for ligaments and muscles of the pelvic floor.

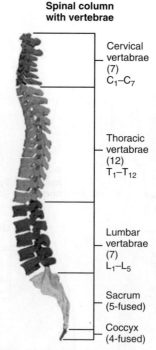

Spinal column with vertebrae

Cervical
vertabrae
(7)
$C_1–C_7$

Thoracic
vertabrae
(12)
$T_1–T_{12}$

Lumbar
vertabrae
(7)
$L_1–L_5$

Sacrum
(5-fused)

Coccyx
(4-fused)

FIGURE 4.9 Divisions of the spinal column.

FOCUS ON READING

Read the following passage and answer the questions that follow.

1. Cancer is a disease that occurs as a result of changes in normal cells. These changes lead to uncontrolled growth that may cause a lump called a tumor except in the case of blood cancer or leukemia. Dr Otto Warburg discovered that cancer is caused by impaired cellular inspiration which means that the cells can no longer use oxygen to burn glucose so that energy is produced. Tumors can be either benign or malignant. Benign tumors do not spread to nearby tissues or to other parts of the body and, in general, these grow at a slow rate and do not constitute a threat to life unless these press on other organs such as the brain or blood vessels. On the other hand, malignant or cancerous tumors usually increase faster and spread from the primary source to other tissues or body parts and destroy them. In other words, malignant tumors can invade their surrounding tissues or organs. Cancer may occur in different body parts. It can affect the blood (leukemia), lungs, pancreas, uterine, brain, breasts, bladder, colon, prostate, etc.

2. Medical reports indicate that lung cancer is the most dangerous of all types of cancers and diseases. Lung cancer kills about 160,000 people a year in the USA alone – more than breast cancer, colon cancer, and prostate cancer combined. The vast majority of cases are smoking related, but **curbing** the use of tobacco is not the only challenge we have. Many nonsmokers also suffer from lung cancer and this raises many questions for oncologists. Why do some smokers stay healthy, but nonsmokers are often affected? Are females more susceptible than males? How effective is early detection of the disease? The National Cancer Institute recently announced a new research plan – and after decades of discouragement, some researchers are voicing cautious optimism. Researchers in genetics are investigating mutations that may make some people vulnerable. Furthermore, biologists and radiologists are devising new ways to detect small, localized tumors, and new treatments are beginning to extend survival times, even for patients in their advanced stages.

3. The etiology of lung cancer is no longer a mystery: some 87% of all cases result directly from smoking. The most effective way to protect yourself from lung cancer, regardless of your gender, age, career, or family history is to quit smoking. Unfortunately, quitting smoking does not entirely remove the damage that tobacco smoke causes to tissues of the lungs. Therefore, former smokers remain more **susceptible** than nonsmokers.

4. In addition to smoking, there are other causes that may lead to cancer. It is often reported that family history is among the major factors that may cause lung cancer. Marshall Anderson from the University of Cincinnati

Medical Center conducted a study to identify susceptibility genes that may cause cancer. He analyzed blood and tissue samples from 52 high-risk families, and traced their shared risk to a small region of human chromosome 6. If labs could be as efficient in this issue as they are now in tests on breast and colon cancer genes, high-risk people could be singled out for special precautions, intensive screening, and possibly even personalized treatments.

5. The challenge that researchers and physicians encounter is to diagnose the disease at an early and treatable stage. Patients early diagnosed with small, localized tumors enjoy a 5-year survival rate of nearly 50%. Lung cancer usually develops silently without causing any of the usual symptoms such as hoarseness, wheezing, coughing, and chest pain. Unfortunately, such symptoms can only be noticed when the tumors are large and dispersed. By the time patients get diagnosed with lung cancer, at least three out of four patients already have reached the stage of metastasis, where the disease has moved from its primary location to other parts of the lung or body. Traditional chest X-rays have never been found effective in increasing survival rates, but experts are now hoping that a new technique – the so-called spiral CT scan (computed tomography, often called helical CT) – will succeed where old methods have failed. The X-ray tube in the CT revolves around the chest and identifies even the tiniest lesions in the tissues of the lung. These CT scans enable doctors to exactly identify the lung tumors and safely **excise** them. Nowadays, oncologist and researchers recommend that high-risk patients should undergo annual CT exams. However, not all health institutions **endorse** routine screening.

6. Although early diagnosis is essential in the process of saving patients' lives, it remains part of the challenge. Although patients diagnosed early enjoy a better chance than those diagnosed late, half of *them* still suffer serious recurrences within 5 years. Fortunately, recent studies revealed that the survival rate may rise up to 70% if traditional chemotherapy is administered after surgery. In the meantime, researchers are still investigating new drugs that may have better life-saving prospects.

A. **Comprehension: Circle the letter of the correct answer.**
   1. Paragraph 1 is mainly about
      a. types of cancer
      b. causes of cancer
      c. types and causes of tumors
      d. treatment of tumors
   2. According to the text, the major cause of cancer is
      a. age
      b. race
      c. family history
      d. smoking

3. According to the text, lung cancer
   a. is easy to detect
   b. is transmitted in the genes
   c. does not show clear signs in its early development
   d. can be easily cured with drugs
4. According to the text, what things are researchers working on to fight cancer
   a. developing new drugs
   b. raising people's awareness of the dangers of smoking
   c. conducting research on genes
   d. all of the above
5. Traditional X-rays were not effective in detecting cancer because they
   a. could not detect very small tumors before they spread
   b. were too dangerous to use often
   c. were too complex to use often
   d. are too expensive
6. According to the text, what is the most important thing that can be done in order to fight cancer?
   a. give money to cancer charities
   b. develop more drugs
   c. get everybody to use the CT scan
   d. stop people from smoking
7. Paragraph 2 is about
   a. cancer statistics
   b. challenges in treating tumors
   c. CT scans
   d. National Cancer Institute
8. Which of the following is not part of the author's purpose in this text?
   a. to get governments to give more money for cancer research
   b. to indicate that genetics can help determine the possibility of getting cancer
   c. to emphasize that smoking is a major cause of cancer
   d. to show that drugs and X-rays do not help much
9. Recent studies indicate that traditional chemotherapy administered after surgery
   a. increases survival chances by 7%
   b. decreases survival chances by 70%
   c. increases survival chances by 70%
   d. has very little effect on survival rates
10. The pronoun *them* in paragraph 6 refers to
    a. all cancer patients
    b. cases where cancer is detected early in its development
    c. cases where cancer is detected late in its development
    d. cases where cancer is hard to treat

11. Which of the following phrases most closely matches the meaning of the phrase "curbing the use of tobacco" in paragraph 2?
    a. increasing the use of tobacco
    b. improving the use of tobacco
    c. controlling the use of tobacco
    d. allowing the use of tobacco

12. In paragraph 5, the phrase " ... safely excise them" means
    a. examine them safely
    b. X-ray them easily
    c. cut them safely
    d. detect them easily

13. In paragraph 5, the verb "endorse" could be replaced with
    a. recommend
    b. acknowledge
    c. deny
    d. evaluate

B. **Find words in the text that mean**
    1. penetrate body tissues (para. 1): _____
    2. vulnerable or easily affected (para. 3): _____
    3. treated differently (para. 4): _____
    4. restricted to a specific body part (para. 5)
    5. happening again (para. 6): _____

C. **Word building: Complete the following table as required.**

Adverb	Adjective	Noun	Verb
		mutation	
xxx	susceptible		xxx
xxx	xxx	inspiration	
xxx		recurrence	
xxx		survival	
xxx			identify
			volunteer
xxx			administer

VOCABULARY DEVELOPMENT

Medical Collocations

Practice 4.6 Fill in the blanks in each of the following sentences with the correct particle from the list. Some particles can be used more than once.

out   up   down   over   of   through   on

1. The nurse **pointed** _____ that the patient took his medicine 2 h ago.
2. Two cardiologists are planning to **carry** _____ an open-heart surgery next week.
3. The doctor advised me to **work** _____ every day in the morning.
4. It is difficult for me to breathe. My nose is **stuffed** _____.
5. My stomach is agitated. I may **throw** _____ anytime.
6. Overweight people must **cut** _____ on fried and fatty foods.
7. Do not come close to me. I think that I am **coming** _____ with a bad flue.
8. My friend will be back at work soon. He has finally **gotten** _____ the stomach virus he had last week.
9. The doctor gave me a strong ointment to **get rid** _____ the rash on my hands and legs.
10. The driver was seriously injured in the accident, but the doctor says he will **pull** _____.
11. The classroom was so hot and stuffy that one of the students **passed** _____.
12. The football player needs to go on a diet. He has put ____ so much weight over the holidays.

Practice 4.7 List the collocations in the previous practice and give their meanings.
1. **Point out:** indicate or specify
2. _____
3. _____
4. _____
5. _____
6. _____
7. _____
8. _____
9. _____
10. _____
11. _____
12. _____

Academic Words

Study the following academic lists.

Academic List 1:

Words	Definitions
1. internal	inside of something (a person's body)
2. confer	to discuss something with other people, so that everyone can express their opinions and decide on something

Words	Definitions
3. cycle	an interval of time during which a characteristic, often regularly repeated event or sequence of events occurs
4. mechanism	a system that is intended to achieve something or deal with a problem
5. principal	first or highest in rank or importance
6. attribute	to regard as arising from a particular cause or source
7. implement	to take action or make changes that you have officially decided should happen
8. code (n)	a set of rules, laws, or principles that tell people how to behave
9. promote	to help something to develop or increase
10. series	a number of objects or events arranged or coming one after the other in succession

Academic List 2:

Words	Definitions
1. investigate	to observe or inquire in detail; examine systematically
2. parameter	a set of fixed limits that control the way that something should be done
3. inadequate	insufficient
4. label (n)	a piece of paper or another material that is attached to something and gives information about it
5. attitude	the opinions and feelings that you usually have about something, especially when this is shown in your behavior
6. prior	existing or arranged before something else or before the present situation
7. stress	continuous feelings of worry about your work or personal life, that prevent you from relaxing
8. implicate	convey a meaning indirectly
9. integrate	to make into a whole by bringing all parts together
10. committed	obligated, or devoted, as by a pledge

Practice 4.8 Match the words in column A with their definitions in column B by writing the letter of the correct answer next to the word in column A.

A	B
1. confer _____	a. convey a meaning indirectly
2. attribute _____	b. an interval of time during which a characteristic, often regularly repeated, event or sequence of events occurs
3. promote _____	c. to discuss something with other people, so that everyone can express their opinions and decide on something
4. stress _____	d. a number of objects or events arranged or coming one after the other in succession
5. attitude _____	e. a set of fixed limits that control the way that something should be done

A	B
6. implicate _____	f. to observe or inquire in detail; examine systematically
7. parameter _____	g. to regard as arising from a particular cause or source
8. series _____	h. continuous feelings of worry about your work or personal life, that prevent you from relaxing
9. cycles _____	i. to help something to develop or increase
10. investigate _____	j. the opinions and feelings that you usually have about something, especially when this is shown in your behavior

Practice 4.9 Complete each of the following sentences using the correct word from the box.

principally	implemented	mechanism	coded	conferred
internally	promotes	cycles	series	attributable

1. The patient is bleeding _____, and needs to be operated on immediately.
2. Thousands of deaths each year are _____ to drunk drivers.
3. I have _____ with your family doctor, and we both feel that an operation is unnecessary at this point.
4. Eating too much sugar _____ tooth decay.
5. The information _____ on DNA must be preserved for the survival of an organism.
6. Harvey is overweight _____ because he does not ever do any exercise.
7. While we sleep, we experience repeated _____ of brain activity.
8. A properly _____ diet can help to improve health and reduce stress.
9. Eating is a requirement for living; therefore, there must be _____ in the body and mind that make us hungry and interested in eating at regular intervals.
10. Psychologists believed that every child goes through a _____ of personality development stages.

Practice 4.10 Complete each of the following sentences using the correct word from the box.

disintegrate	prior	inadequate	attitude	implicated
label	parameter	stress	committed	investigating

The scientific method is the main tool used by psychologists for _____ both the mind and behavior.

1. Dr Hans Selye observed that adopting the right attitude can convert a negative _____ into a positive one.
2. Recent research suggests that children born to teenage mothers are more likely to be poor, and to receive _____ health care and education.
3. Evidence suggests that newborn babies can hear and remember things which occurred _____ to birth.
4. Stress has been _____ in a wide variety of illnesses.
5. According to the information on the _____, you should take this medication just before meal time.
6. After analyzing the available medical data, doctors decided to modify the original _____ of the spreadsheet to accommodate more information.
7. Our company policy states that we are _____ to fairness and honesty in all our dealings.
8. Human hair and fingernails are the last part of the body to _____ after we die.
9. Many psychologists believe that we form our _____ and opinions of ourselves in part by observing our own behavior.

FOCUS ON GRAMMAR

Confusing Verbs

Some verbs in English are troublesome and confusing to students in terms of meaning and spelling such as the verbs *lie* and *lay*. A brief description of the meanings and forms of these verbs may be helpful.

Present	Past	Past Participle	Present Participle	Meaning
lie	lay	lain	lying	recline on a horizontal or resting position, occupy a position or place
lie	lied	lied	lying	present false information
lay	laid	laid	laying	place, produce eggs

Examples

The farmer was very tired and so he lay under a tree to take a nap.
I have lain on the bed for half an hour.
I laid the book on the table.
He lied to me when I asked him why he was absent.
Our house lies behind that the police station.

Practice 4.11 Fill in the blank in each of the following sentences with the correct form of the verbs: *lie* or *lay*. State whether the action means recline, place, or give false information.

1. The patient has _____ in bed all day.
   Meaning: _____.
2. Where did the lab technician _____ his lab coat?
   Meaning: _____
3. These medications _____ on this table last week.
   Meaning: _____
4. The old man was _____ down when the doctor came to see him.
5. These X-rays do not _____. They are usually accurate.
   Meaning: _____
6. Our college _____ on the side of the river between those trees.
   Meaning: _____

Practice 4.12 Use each of the confusing verbs in the list above in a sentence of your own.

1. lie: _____ (recline)
2. lie: _____ (occupy a position)
3. lay: _____(place/put)
4. lie: _____ (present false information)

ORAL COMMUNICATION SKILLS

Role play: Doctor–patient conversation
1. Work with a partner and complete the dialogue between a doctor and his patient.
   Dr Sami: Good morning Mr Ali.
   Ali: _____
   Dr Sami: What's wrong with you?
   Ali: _____
   Dr Sami: Do you suffer from any other problem?
   Ali: _____

Dr Sami: Let me check you fever and feel your pulse. Don't worry. Everything is normal. There is nothing serious. I will give you two medicines. One is a painkiller and the other is for allergy. You will feel much better in a couple of days.

Ali: _____

Dr Sami: However, you need to get your blood tested for hemoglobin. Bring me the report tomorrow in the afternoon.

Ali: _____

Dr Sami: I will give you a sick leave for 2 days. You need to relax.

Ali: Thank you doctor. Can you tell me how to take the medicines?

Dr Sami: _____

Ali: What should I eat doctor? Any special food?

Dr Sami: _____

Ali: Thank you doctor. See you tomorrow.

1. Act out the dialogue.
2. Summarize the reading passage orally in your own words.

FOCUS ON WRITING

Practice 4.13 Write an extended definition for one of the following items:

1. Body positions
2. Body planes
3. Body cavities

REVIEW EXERCISES

A. **Case study 1:** Read the following case study and answer the questions following it.

A 65-year-old man who recently retired from his work as an architect was admitted to an accident and emergency department (A&E) because of intermittent pain in the chest for 3 days. He was a chronic smoker for more than 25 years with a history of hypertension in addition to feelings of discomfort, pressure, heaviness, or pain in arm. An ECG was done at the emergency department which revealed that the patient suffers from an anterior ST-elevation myocardial infarction (STEMI). Therefore, thrombolysis was given due to the persistent chest pain in order to dissolve clots in blood vessels, improve blood flow, and prevent damage to tissues and organs. A loading dose of aspirin, clopidogrel, and enoxaparin were administered as well. He was then sent to the CCU where his blood pressure dropped to 70/49 mm Hg and his pulse rose up to 120/min. He was sweating profusely but his temperature was still within normal range. Physical examination revealed an elevated JVP together with a pansystolic murmur throughout the precordium. The ECG did not show any serial change.

Answer the following questions:

1. Why was the old man taken to hospital?
2. Describe his history.
3. How was his health problem diagnosed?
4. What was the diagnosis?
5. Why was he given thrombolysis?
6. Find a word in the text that is the opposite of *posterior*.
7. Find a word in the text that means *discontinuous*.
8. What do the abbreviations ECG, CCU, JVP stand for?
9. Find a word that means continuous.
10. Give the noun forms of prevent, retire, persistent.
11. Define the phrase "a loading dose"?

Case study 2: Read the following case study and answer the questions following it.

June 26, 2016

Ayman Muaz, MD

210 University City Street

Sharjah, UAE 10669

RE: Karima Ali

DOB: 1/03/55

1. Mrs Karima was seen in consultation for further evaluation and treatment of a right first rib and clavicular problem. She is a 61-year-old female who had developed significant right anterior chest wall pain in the parasternal area higher up. This occurred for the first time in March of 2015. The pain improved and became much less problematic. The patient notices a worsening pain when she has a spell of coughing or with deep breathing. There is some radiation to the axilla.
2. The patient has a history of trauma to the right shoulder while lifting weights. **This** caused a chronic pain in the shoulder for quite a few years and was finally diagnosed as a separated shoulder back in 2010 and was treated with a distal clavicle resection and an acromioplasty. She does have

a history of a preview X-ray done in 2012 which showed a bony abnormality at this same spot. The patient has had a workup of this with a bone scan done on May 19, 2013, which showed abnormal tracer activity in the medial right clavicle or the medial right first rib corresponding to the osseous area on the chest X-ray. This was felt to represent hypertrophic changes with bridging of the medial right clavicle on the first rib. The patient also had a CT scan of the chest which showed an osseous abnormality at the junction of the right first rib and clavicle done on May 16, 2013. This had a benign appearance. The patient denies any recent trauma to the chest or shoulder.

3. Physical examination: The patient is a thin, 61-year-old female. Her vital signs show a blood pressure of 128/80, pulse of 80, and respiratory rate of 16. Her neck exam shows no cervical adenopathy and her thyroid is normal. Her heart exam has a regular rate and rhythm and no murmurs. Her lungs have clear breath sounds bilaterally. Her right clavicular area is not prominent visually and is not tender by palpation. There is some tenderness in the right parasternal area at about the third rib. Otherwise, the patient has normal breast development and normal chest contour. The abdomen is flat and not tender with no hepatomegaly. The extremities have good range of motion. There are palpable peripheral pulses and no peripheral edema. The neuromuscular exam shows grossly intact strength and sensation in all extremities and the cranial nerves are intact bilaterally. The patient is oriented to person, place, and time.

4. My impression is that the patient appears to have a process involving the right first rib and clavicle with ossification indicating a chronic problem. I suspect this is related to her history of previous right shoulder trauma with weightlifting about 6 years ago. I see no evidence of a soft tissue tumor and the bony appearance, as mentioned in the CT report, appears benign. This may be related to her recent history of pain, although I think a conservative approach is in order. I would recommend a follow-up CT scan in 3 months. She should treat the pain symptomatically and resort to narcotics only if necessary. I see no need for an invasive biopsy at this time.

Find a word in the case study that means

1. further _____
2. front _____
3. middle _____
4. pertaining to skull _____
5. pertaining to the neck _____
6. any disease of a gland _____

7. pertaining to both sides _____
8. armpit _____
9. The term "parasternal" means
   a. above the sternum
   b. below the sternum
   c. near the sternum
   d. behind the sternum
10. The word clavicular mostly means:
   a. either of the bones joining the breastbone to the shoulder blades
   b. breastbone
   c. muscle
   d. shoulder blades
11. Write T or F after each statement
   a. The patient's chief complaint was attributed to radiation. _____
   b. Dr Ayman recommended that the patient take painkillers once a day before bedtime. _____
   c. The patient complains of an acute ossification problem in the first right rib. _____
   d. The physical examination showed that the patient's muscular system had no abnormalities. _____
   e. Upon examination, the patient was found to have an enlarged liver. _____
   f. Acromioplasty is given in the report as part of the patient's past medical history. _____
12. The demonstrative pronoun "this" in paragraph 2 refers to
   a. lifting weights
   b. trauma to the right shoulder
   c. radiation to axilla
   d. coughing and breathing
13. The word "tender" in the text means
   a. soft
   b. painless
   c. painful
   d. abnormal

B. Provide the meaning of each of the following medical terms.

Combining Form	Meaning	Medical Term	Meaning
anter/o	front	anterior _____	
caud/o	tail	caudal _____	
cephal/o	head	cephalic _____	
cervic/o	neck	cervical _____	

Combining Form	Meaning	Medical Term	Meaning
chondr/o	cartilage	hypochondriac _____	
coccyg/o	tailbone	coccygeal _____	
crani/o	skull	cranial _____	
femor/o	thighbone	femoral _____	
infer/o	lower	inferior _____	
inguin/o	groin	inguinal _____	
later/o	side	lateral _____	
lumb/o	loin	lumbar _____	
medi/o	middle	medial _____	
mediastin/o	space between the lungs	mediastinum _____	
pelv/o	hipbone	pelvic _____	
peritone/o	double membrane surrounding the abdomen	Peritoneal _____	
pleur/o	double membrane surrounding each lung	pleural _____	
proxim/o	nearer	proximal _____	
sacr/o	lower back	sacrum _____	
spin/o	vertebral column	spinal _____	
thorac/o	chest	thoracic _____	
trache/o	windpipe	tracheostomy _____	
umbilic/o	navel	umbilical _____	

C. Match the words in column A with their meanings in column B.

A	B
1. abdominopelvic _____	a. pertaining to the sole of the foot
2. adduction _____	b. tailbone
3. cervical _____	c. ventral cavity that contains heart and associated structure
4. coccyx _____	d. toward the surface of the body
5. deep _____	e. lying horizontal with face down
6. eversion _____	f. turning outward
7. inferior _____	g. nearer to the center
8. inversion _____	h. ventral cavity that contains digestive and other structures
9. lumbar _____	i. turning inward

A	B
10. plantar _____	j. neck
11. posterior _____	k. movement toward the median plane
12. prone _____	l. away from the head; toward the tail
13. proximal _____	m. away from the surface of the body
14. superficial _____	n. loin
15. thoracic _____	o. near the back of the body

D. Circle the letter of the most appropriate answer.
  1. Which of the following does not describe the anatomic position?
     a. face forward
     b. arms at side
     c. feet parallel
     d. palms toward the back
  2. The abdominopelvic cavity is separated from the thoracic cavity by the
     a. hipbone
     b. lungs
     c. diaphragm
     d. pelvis
  3. The ventral cavity consists of the
     a. abdominopelvic and thoracic cavities
     b. superior and inferior cavities
     c. thoracic and abdominal cavities
     d. thoracic and spinal cavities
  4. The peritoneum is
     a. the large membrane that lines the abdominopelvic cavity
     b. the membrane around the lungs
     c. the large membrane that lines the thoracic cavity
     d. the membrane around the heart
  5. A dorsal structure is located
     a. toward the back
     b. toward the front
     c. toward the midline
     d. toward the side
  6. The opposite of distal is
     a. inferior
     b. lateral
     c. proximal
     d. anterior
  7. A term that means the same as posterior is
     a. dorsal
     b. inferior
     c. cephalic
     d. ventral

8. The opposite of inferior is
   a. distal
   b. dorsal
   c. medial
   d. superior

9. The elbow is proximal to the
   a. shoulder
   b. arm
   c. wrist
   d. neck

10. A person in a supine position is
    a. sitting
    b. lying face up
    c. standing and looking forward
    d. lying face down

11. The opposite of supine is
    a. prone
    b. superior
    c. pronated
    d. prognathic

12. A transverse plane divides the body into
    a. ventral and dorsal
    b. anterior and posterior parts
    c. right and left parts
    d. superior and inferior parts

13. A frontal plane divides the body into
    a. superior and inferior parts
    b. anterior and posterior parts
    c. left and right parts
    d. lateral parts

14. The cranial cavity is a subdivision of the
    a. abdominal cavity
    b. pelvic cavity
    c. dorsal cavity
    d. ventral cavity

15. The most superior medial region of the abdomen is the
    a. epigastric
    b. iliac
    c. lumbar
    d. hypochondriac

16. The central, medial region of the abdomen is the
    a. umbilical
    b. right lumbar
    c. left hypochondriac
    d. hypogastric

17. The region of the abdomen that contains the hip bone is the
   a. lumbar
   b. right hypochondriac
   c. epigastric
   d. iliac
18. The abbreviations LUQ, RUQ, RLQ, and LLQ refer to
   a. quadrants of the abdomen
   b. regions of the heart
   c. the dorsal body cavity
   d. the arms and legs
19. The term *coccygeal* refers to the
   a. tailbone
   b. diaphragm
   c. buttocks
   d. liver
20. *Cervicobrachial* refers to the
   a. hand and foot
   b. neck and spine
   c. brain and face
   d. neck and arm
21. Podiatry is a specialty for the study and treatment of the
   a. lung
   b. skin
   c. eyes
   d. foot
22. The antebrachium is the
   a. shoulder
   b. forearm
   c. wrist
   d. elbow
23. The etiology of a disease is its
   a. outcome
   b. severity
   c. cause
   d. immune response

E. Match the proper anatomical term in column A with the common term in column B for the body regions listed below.

A	B
1 inguinal _____	a. breastbone
2 frontal _____	b. sole
3 sternal _____	c. armpit
4 carpal _____	d. toe

A	B
5 gluteal _____	e. base of skull
6 antecubital _____	f. point of shoulder
7 plantar _____	g. shoulder blade
8 digital _____	h. groin
9 scapular _____	i. buttock
10 popliteal _____	j. cheek
11 axillary _____	k. thumb
12 acromial _____	l. wrist
13 occipital _____	m. back of knee
14 pollex _____	n. forehead
15 buccal _____	o. front of elbow

F. **Label each numbered part. Write its name in the table below.**

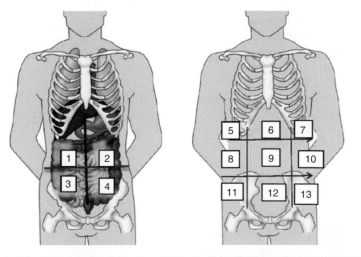

	Name
1	
2	
3	
4	
5	
6	
7	
8	
9	
10	
11	
12	
13	

G. **Complete each of the following sentences using the proper term from the box.**

| anterior | posterior | inferior | proximal | lateral |
| distal | superficial | deep | superior | medial |

1. The forehead is _____ to the nose.
2. The navel is _____ to the breastbone.
3. The breastbone is _____ to the spine.
4. The heart is _____ to the arm.
5. The elbow is _____ to the wrist.
6. The heart is _____ to the breastbone.
7. The knee is _____ to the thigh.
8. The skin is _____ to the skeleton.
9. The lungs are _____ to the rib cage.
10. The arms are _____ to the chest.

H. **Name the body parts that refer to the following adjectives.**

1. phalangeal _____
2. cervical _____
3. intercostal _____
4. macrocephaly _____
5. sublingual _____
6. syndactyly _____
7. circumoral _____
8. periosteum _____
9. infraumbilical _____
10. bipedal _____

I. **Label each body position. Write its name below the figure.**

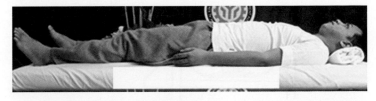

1. _____

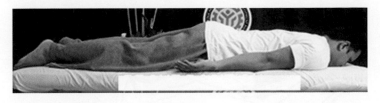

2. _____

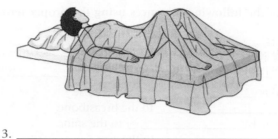

3. _____

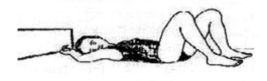

4. _____

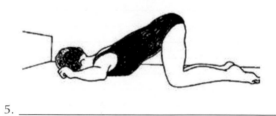

5. _____

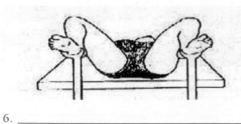

6. _____

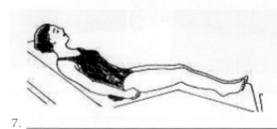

7. _____

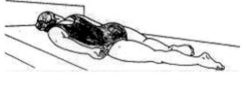

8. _____

J. **Identify the root in each of the following terms and define it.**

Term	Root	Meaning of Root
1. polymorphous	_____	_____
2. jaundice	_____	_____
3. visceral	_____	_____
4. somatic	_____	_____
5. femoral	_____	_____
6. antebrachium	_____	_____
7. cirrhosis	_____	_____
8. heterochromic	_____	_____
9. inferior	_____	_____
10. caudal	_____	_____

K. **Circle the correct answer.**

1. Which bone is also known as the thighbone?
      a. tibia   b. femur   c. patella   d. sternum
2. Pertaining to the tailbone is termed
      a. cervical   b. sacral   c. coccygeal   d. thoracic
3. The combining form for flesh tissue is
      a. sacr/o   b. thromb/o   c. gynec/o   d. sarc/o
4. Pertaining to the area between the lungs in the chest is termed
      a. diaphragm   b. mediastinal   c. thoracic   d. epithelial
5. The plane that divides the body into upper and lower portions is
      a. cervical   b. frontal   c. transverse   d. sagittal
6. The four fused bones at the end of the spinal column are
      a. coccygeal bones   b. lumbar bones
      c. sacral bones   d. cervical bones
7. A backbone is called
      a. disk   b. vertebra   c. cartilage   d. vertebrae
8. The backbones in the region of the waist are
      a. lumbar bones   b. cervical bones
      c. coccygeal bones   d. sacral bones
9. The patella is also called
      a. shin bone   b. breastbone   c. thighbone   d. kneecap

10. The ileum is part of the
    a. abdominal cavity   b. chest cavity
    c. pelvic cavity   d. dorsal cavity

SELF-ASSESSMENT

Check (✓) what you learned. If you need more information or practice, refer to the relevant section in the chapter.

( ) I can differentiate between the levels of body organization.
( ) I can identify combining forms and tell their meanings.
( ) I can name the major body systems and their functions.
( ) I can analyze medical terms pertaining to body structure into their constituents.
( ) I can identify body planes and regions.
( ) I can identify body positions.
( ) I can identify body cavities and the organs within each.
( ) I can identify directional terms.
( ) I can use certain medical collocations and academic words properly.
( ) I can pronounce medical terms properly.
( ) I can read medical texts for main ideas and details.
( ) I can ask and answer questions pertaining to medical issues.
( ) I can report medical cases orally.
( ) I can spell the new medical terms in the chapter.

CHAPTER 5

Body Systems

LEARNING OUTCOMES

At the end of this chapter, students are expected to:

1. differentiate between the terms system, organ, and tissue
2. identify body systems
3. identify the body organs in each system
4. explain the major functions of each system
5. identify and define the roots and medical terms pertaining to each system
6. interpret abbreviations used in reference to each system
7. pronounce new medical terms pertaining to each system
8. write a referral letter
9. use new words and medical terms in daily activities

CONTENTS

BODY SYSTEMS

The human body is very complex because it consists of a huge number of microscopic parts that have their own special properties. They work together in a very delicate and well-organized manner to best serve the human being. These small structures are the cells, tissues, organs, and systems.

The cell is the basic structural, functional, and simplest unit of any living organism. Cells can maintain life and reproduce themselves. Each cell consists of cytoplasm and a nucleus enclosed in a membrane. The human body, which starts as a single, newly fertilized cell, consists of a great number of cells. These small cells are grouped together in a highly organized manner in order to form tissues. This means that a tissue is a structure of a great number of similar cells. Tissues can be of different types: muscle, connective, epithelial, and nervous.

Organs, on the other hand, are far more complex than tissues. An organ or a body part consists of tissues that perform one or more specific functions.

Organs of the body include the heart, the liver, the stomach, the eye, the nose, the kidney, and the ear, etc.

Finally, a system consists of varying numbers and types of organs that perform complex functions. Systems do not function in isolation of each other. Their functions are inextricably tied to each other. No system can function independently. The body systems work together to form an organism or a living thing such as a plant, bacterium, fungus, or an animal.

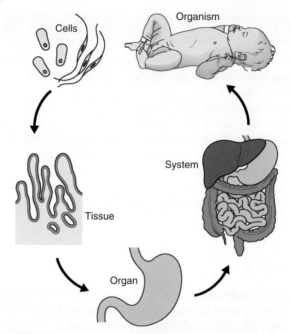

FIGURE 5.1 Images for cells, tissues, organs, systems, and organisms.

The following are the major types of body systems:

1. The **integumentary system** includes the skin and its appendages such as the hair, nails, sweat, and oil glands. The skin is the largest body organ. It protects the body from various kinds of damage, such as loss of water or abrasion from outside. The skin performs the following functions:
   - provides a physical barrier against microorganisms and foreign materials
   - prevents absorption of harmful substances from outside the body
   - protects underlying structures, such as fragile organs
   - protects against excessive sun exposure (ultraviolet rays)

- cushions internal organs against trauma
- produces secretions for protection and water regulation
- absorbs helpful medicines
- communicates feelings and moods through facial expressions
- prevents nutrients from being washed out of the body
- controls body temperature by convection, evaporation, conduction, and radiation

It is obvious now that the skin performs protection, thermoregulation, metabolism, sensation, communication, and perspiration.

The skin is divided into a number of layers. The **epidermis** is the thin superficial layer. It is the outermost protective layer of the skin. The second layer that comes below the epidermis is called the **dermis.** It is thicker than the epidermis and contains collagen and elastin – fibers that give strength, structure, and elasticity.

The third layer is the **subcutaneous** layer that consists of mainly fat and it is the source of nerves and blood vessels as well as the roots of your hair follicles, oil glands, and sweat glands.

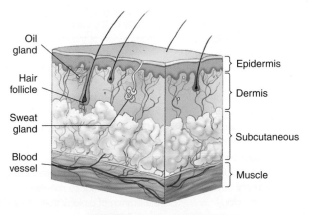

FIGURE 5. 2 Layers of the skin.

Table 5.1 Roots for the Integumentary System

Root	Meaning	Example	Meaning
adip/o	fat	adiposis	abnormal condition of fatty tissue in the body
ambly/o	dull, dim	amblyopia	dimness of vision
audi/o	hearing	audiometer	instrument for measuring hearing

Continued

Table 5.1 Roots for the Integumentary System—Cont'd

Root	Meaning	Example	Meaning
aur/o auricul/o	hearing	aural auriculocranial	■ pertaining to hearing ■ pertaining to the auricle of the ear and cranium
blephar/o	eyelid	blepharoptosis	drooping of the eyelids
cerumin/o	wax	ceruminolytic	agent for softening earwax
choroid/o	choroid (the dark-brown vascular coat of the eye between the sclera and the retina)	subchoroidal	below the choroid
cochle/o	cochlea	cochleitis	inflammation of the cochlea
conjunctiv/o	conjunctiva	conjunctivoplasty	plastic surgery of the conjunctiva
core/o	pupil	coreoplasty	surgical correction of the size and shape of the pupil
corne/o	cornea	corneoblepharon	adhesion of the eyelid margin to the cornea
cutane/o	skin	subcutaneous	pertaining to beneath the skin
cycl/o	ciliary body	cyclodialysis	method of relieving intraocular pressure in glaucoma
dacry/o	tears	dacryorrhea	an excessive secretion of tears
derm/o dermat/o	skin	dermal dermatology	■ pertaining to the skin ■ study of the skin
hidr/o	sweat	hidradenitis	inflammation of the sweat glands
ichthy/o	dry, scaly	ichthyosis	abnormal condition of dry skin
irid/o	iris	iridocele	herniation of a portion of the iris through a corneal defect
kerat/o	horny layer of the skin	keratolysis	separation of the horny layer of the skin
labyrinth/o	inner ear	labyrinthitis	inflammation of the inner ear
lacrim/o	tears	lacrimotomy	incision into the lacrimal duct
lent/i	lens	lentiform	resembling a lens
lip/o	fat	lipocele	hernia containing fat
mastoid/o	mastoid	mastoiditis	inflammation of the mastoid process
melan/o	dark, black	melanocyte	a cell that produces melanin
myc/o	fungus	mycology	the branch of biology that deals with fungi
myring/o	eardrum	myringotomy	incision of the eardrum
nas/o	nose	nasal	pertaining to the nose
ocul/o	eye	ocular	pertaining to the eye
onych/o	nail	onychomalacia	softening of the nails
ophthalm/o	eye	ophthalmologist	specialist in the study and treatment of the eye
opt/o	eye	optometer	instrument for determining eye refraction
ossicul/o	ossicle (a small bone, especially one of the three bones of the middle ear)	ossiculectomy	excision of one of the ossicles in the middle ear
ot/o	ear	otitis	inflammation of the ear
palpebr/o	eyelid	palpebral	pertaining to the eyelid

Table 5.1 Roots for the Integumentary System—Cont'd

Root	Meaning	Example	Meaning
phak/o	lens of the eye	aphakia	absence of the lens of the eye
pil/o	hair	pilonidal	pertaining to hair in a cyst
pupill/o	pupil	iridopupillary	pertaining to the iris and the pupil
retin/o	retina	retinitis	inflammation of the retina
rhin/o	nose	rhinitis	inflammation of the nose
salping/o	auditory tube	salpingoscope	instrument to examine the Eustachian tubes
scler/o	whiting of the eye	sclerectasia	protrusion of the sclera
scot/o	darkness	scotometer	instrument for evaluation of blind spot
seb/o	sebum	seborrhea	excess flow of sebum
steat/o	fat	steatosis	the abnormal accumulation of fat within a cell or organ
sudor/o	sweat	sudoresis	profuse sweating
trich/o	hair	trichophagia	compulsive eating of hair
tympan/o	eardrum	tympanoplasty	plastic repair of the eardrum
ungu/o	nail	ungual	pertaining to the nails
uve/o	uvea (the vascular middle layer of the eye)	uveitis	inflammation of the uvea
vestibul/o	vestibule (entrance to another body) cavity)	vestibulotomy	incision of the vestibule of the inner ear
xen/o	foreign	xenograft	skin transplantation from a foreign donor
xer/o	dry	xeroderma	dryness of the skin

Practice 5.1 Use the root **onych/o** to form words that mean:

1. tumors of the nails _____
2. softening of the nails _____
3. abnormal condition of the nails _____
4. abnormal condition of the nails caused by fungus _____
5. abnormal condition of a hidden nail _____
6. disease of the nails _____

Practice 5.2 Identify the root in each of the following terms and define it.

Term	Root	Meaning of Root
1. hypodermis	_____	_____
2. eponychium	_____	_____
3. hypertrichosis	_____	_____
4. keratosis	_____	_____
5. hidradenitis	_____	_____
6. adipectomy	_____	_____
7. lipocele	_____	_____
8. dermatoplasty	_____	_____

Practice 5.3 Match each of the following terms in column A with its meaning in column B.

A	B
1 conjunctiva _____	a. pertaining to hair in a cyst
2 sclera _____	b. outer layer of the skin
3 subungual _____	c. malignant tumor of pigmented cells in the skin
4 epidermis _____	d. absence of the lens of the eye
5 myringotomy _____	e. any disease of the retina
6 melanoma _____	f. visual examination of the ear
7 otoscopy _____	g. white, outer coat of the eyeball
8 aphakia _____	h. pertaining to under the nail
9 retinopathy _____	i. incision into the eardrum
10 pilonidal _____	j. thin, protective membrane over the front of the eye

Table 5.2 Abbreviations Used for the Integumentary System

Abbreviation	Meaning
AD	right ear
AS	left ear
ENT	ear, nose, throat
HEENT	head, eyes, ears, nose, throat
HL	hearing level
ID	intradermal
IOL	intraocular lens
IOP	intraocular pressure
IV	intravenous
NVA	near visual acuity
OD	right eye
OS	left eye
OT	otolaryngology
OU	both eyes/each eye
PERRLA	pupils equal, round, reactive to light and accommodation
ST	speech threshold
TM	tympanic membrane
VA	visual acuity
VF	visual fields
XP	xeroderma pigmentosum

2. The **musculoskeletal system** consists of all the bones of the body (206) and their associated cartilages, muscles, tendons, ligaments, and joints. This system provides form, stability, and support to the body. It also enables the body to move. The body bones work with the muscles in order to maintain the body positions and to produce controlled and precise movements.

The skeleton performs five major functions:

- provides structural support and framework for the body.
- stores minerals and lipids: most of the calcium the body needs is stored in the bones; the bones also store energy reserves as lipid in areas filled with yellow marrow.
- produces blood cells: red blood cells, white blood cells, and other blood elements are produced in the red marrow which fills the internal cavities of many bones; blood production is called hematopoiesis.
- protects the body organs: many soft tissues and organs are surrounded by skeletal elements; for example, the rib cage protects the heart and lungs; the skull protects the brain; the vertebrae protect the spinal cord; and the pelvis protects the delicate reproductive organs.
- provides control and movement: many bones function as levers that can change the magnitude and direction of the forces generated by muscles.

The skeleton consists of the following main bones:

- The skull: cranium, mandible, and maxilla
- Shoulder girdle: clavicle and scapula
- Arm: humerus, radius, and ulna
- Hand: carpals, metacarpals, and phalanges
- Chest : sternum and ribs
- Spine: cervical area (top 7 vertebrae), thoracic (next 12), lumbar (bottom 5 vertebrae), sacrum (5 fused or stuck together bones), and coccyx (the tiny bit at the bottom of the spine)
- Pelvic girdle: ilium, pubis, and ischium
- Leg: femur, tibia, and fibula
- Ankle: talus and calcaneus
- Foot: tarsals, metatarsals, and phalanges

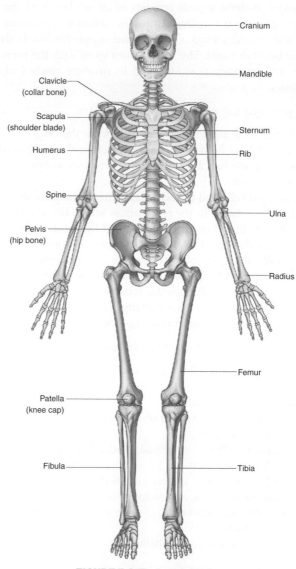

Cranium

Mandible

Clavicle
(collar bone)

Scapula
(shoulder blade)

Sternum

Humerus

Rib

Spine

Ulna

Pelvis
(hip bone)

Radius

Femur

Patella
(knee cap)

Fibula

Tibia

FIGURE 5.3 The human skeleton.

The musculoskeletal system also contains other elements such as:

- **Joints:** These are the structures where two bones are joined.
- **Tendons:** A tendon is a flexible but inelastic cord or fibrous tissue that connects a muscle to a bone.
- **Ligaments:** A ligament is a band of fibrous tissue connecting bones or cartilages.
- **Skeletal muscles:** These muscles contract to pull on tendons and move the bones of the skeleton. These also maintain posture and body position, support soft tissues, guard entrances and exits to the digestive and urinary tracts, and maintain body temperature.
- **Nerves:** Nerves control the contraction of skeletal muscles, interpret sensory information, and coordinate the activities of the organ systems of the body.
- **Cartilage:** This is a type of connective tissue. The body contains three major types of cartilage: hyaline cartilage, elastic cartilage, and fibrocartilage.

LATERAL VIEW

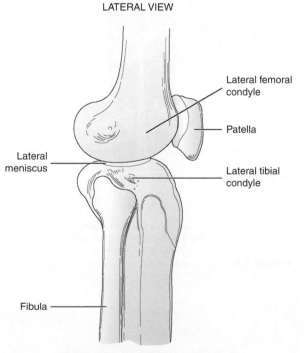

Lateral femoral condyle

Patella

Lateral meniscus

Lateral tibial condyle

Fibula

FIGURE 5.4 Parts of the skeletal system.

There are about 700 muscles in the body. Skeletal muscles are the only muscles in the body that are consciously controlled. The remaining muscles work involuntarily and they are inside the organs of the body such as the heart and the stomach. The skeletal muscles attach two bones together with tendons, which are very strong and can hold up under extreme stress. Muscles lengthen and shorten in order to allow motion so the two bones can move further apart or closer together.

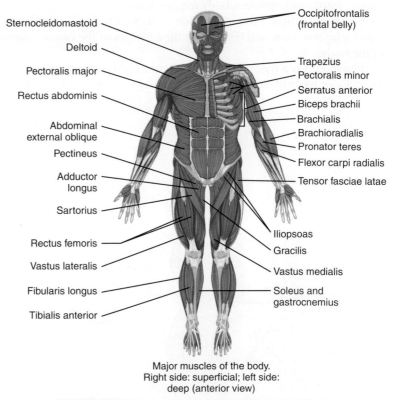

Sternocleidomastoid

Deltoid

Pectoralis major

Rectus abdominis

Abdominal external oblique

Pectineus

Adductor longus

Sartorius

Rectus femoris

Vastus lateralis

Fibularis longus

Tibialis anterior

Occipitofrontalis (frontal belly)

Trapezius

Pectoralis minor

Serratus anterior

Biceps brachii

Brachialis

Brachioradialis

Pronator teres

Flexor carpi radialis

Tensor fasciae latae

Iliopsoas

Gracilis

Vastus medialis

Soleus and gastrocnemius

Major muscles of the body.
Right side: superficial; left side:
deep (anterior view)

FIGURE 5.5 Major muscles of the body (anterior and posterior view).

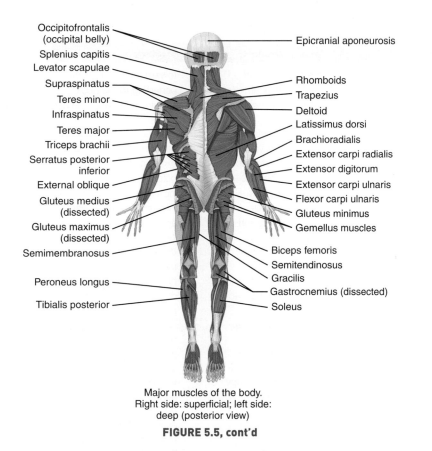

Occipitofrontalis
(occipital belly)
Splenius capitis
Levator scapulae
Supraspinatus
Teres minor
Infraspinatus
Teres major
Triceps brachii
Serratus posterior
inferior
External oblique
Gluteus medius
(dissected)
Gluteus maximus
(dissected)
Semimembranosus
Peroneus longus
Tibialis posterior

Epicranial aponeurosis
Rhomboids
Trapezius
Deltoid
Latissimus dorsi
Brachioradialis
Extensor carpi radialis
Extensor digitorum
Extensor carpi ulnaris
Flexor carpi ulnaris
Gluteus minimus
Gemellus muscles
Biceps femoris
Semitendinosus
Gracilis
Gastrocnemius (dissected)
Soleus

Major muscles of the body.
Right side: superficial; left side:
deep (posterior view)

FIGURE 5.5, cont'd

Table 5.3 Roots for the Musculoskeletal System			
Root	**Meaning**	**Example**	**Meaning**
acetabul/o	the cup-shaped cavity at the base of the hipbone	acetabulectomy	excision of the acetabulum
acromi/o	projection of scapula	acromial	pertaining to the acromion
ankyl/o	stiffness	ankylosis	abnormal condition of stiffness
arthr/o	joint	arthritis	inflammation of the joints
brachi/o	arm	brachialgia	pain in the arm
burs/o	bursa (sacs of fluid near a joint)	peribursal	around a bursa
calcane/o	heel bone	calcaneodynia	pain in the heel
carp/o	wrist bone	carpoptosis	wrist drop

Continued

Table 5.3 Roots for the Musculoskeletal System—Cont'd

Root	Meaning	Example	Meaning
cephal/o	head	cephalad	toward the head
cervic/o	neck	cervical	pertaining to the neck
chondr/o	cartilage	subchondriac	pertaining to under the cartilage of the ribs
clavicul/o	collar bone	clavicular	pertaining to the collar bone
coccyg/o	coccyx (tailbone)	coccygeal	pertaining to the tailbone
condyl/o	knob/end of a bone	condylectomy	excision of the condyle
cost/o	rib	subcostal	below the ribs
crani/o	skull	craniotomy	incision into the skull
dactyl/o	fingers, toes	dactylitis	inflammation of the fingers or toes
erg/o	work	ergograph	an instrument for measuring muscle work
fasci/o	fascia	fasciodesis	binding of a fascia to a tendon
femor/o	femur (thigh bone)	femoral	pertaining to the thigh bone
fibul/o	smaller bone of lower leg	fibulocalcaneal	pertaining to the fibula and calcaneus
humer/o	upper arm bone	humeroscapular	pertaining to the humerus and scapula
ili/o	ilium	iliac	pertaining to the ilium
in/o	fiber	inosclerosis	hardening of tissue from an increase of fiber
ischi/o	lower portion of hipbone	ischiodynia	pain in the ischium
kin/o	movement	kinesis	▪ movement
kinesi/o		kinesitherapy	▪ treatment of movement
kyph/o	humpback	kyphosis	abnormal condition of humpback posture
lamin/o	part of vertebral arch	laminectomy	excision of the lamina to relieve pressure
leiomy/o	smooth muscle	leiomyoma	tumor of smooth muscle
ligament/o	ligament	ligamentous	pertaining to the ligament
lord/o	curve	lordosis	abnormal condition of swayback posture
lumb/o	lower back	lumbar	pertaining to the lower back
maxilla/o	upper jaw	maxillofacial	pertaining to the jaws and face
metacarp/o	handbones	metacarpectomy	excision of the metacarpal
muscul/o	muscle	muscular	pertaining to the muscle
my/o	muscle	myocardial	pertaining to heart muscle
myel/o	bone marrow	myelitis	inflammation of the spinal cord
myos/o	muscle	myositis	inflammation of the muscle
orth/o	straight	orthopedist	specialist in the study and treatment of musculoskeletal order
oste/o	bone	osteoma	a benign tumor of bone tissue
patell/o	kneecap	patellectomy	excision of the kneecap
ped/o	foot	pedograph	instrument for recording the foot

Table 5.3 Roots for the Musculoskeletal System—Cont'd

Root	Meaning	Example	Meaning
pelv/o pelvi/o	hipbone	suprapelvic pelvioscope	▪ above the hipbone ▪ instrument to visually examine the hipbone
phalang/o	bones of fingers and toes	phalangeal	pertaining to fingers and toes
pod/o	foot	podiatry	medical care and treatment of the foot
pub/o	anterior part of pelvic bone	pubococcygeal	pertaining to the pubis and the coccyx
rachi/o	spine	rachiocentesis	surgical puncture of the spine
rhabd/o rhabdomy/o	rod shaped	rhabdoid rhabdomyoma	▪ resembling a rod ▪ tumor composed of striated muscular tissue
sacr/o	sacrum	perisacral	around the sacrum
scoli/o	bent	scoliosis	abnormal condition of the spine
spondyl/o	spinal column	spondylosis	abnormal condition of the vertebra/spinal degeneration
stern/o	breastbone	sternad	toward the sternum
synov/i	membrane	asynovia	lack of synovial fluid
ten/o	tendon	tenodesis	binding of the tendon
tendin/o	tendon	tendinitis	inflammation of the tendon
thorac/o	chest	thoracoschisis	splitting of the chest
tibi/o	tibia (larger bone of lower leg)	tibiafemoral	pertaining to the tibia and femur
ton/o	tone	dystonia	abnormal muscle tone
uln/o	ulna (the bone extending from the elbow to the wrist)	ulnocarpal	pertaining to the ulna and wrist
vertebr/o	vertebra	intervertebral	between the vertebrae

Practice 5.4 Match each of the following terms in column A with its meaning in column B.

A	B
1 intervertebral _____	a. abnormal large head
2 craniotomy _____	b. excision of the patella
3 myelodysplasia _____	c. breastbone
4 sternum _____	d. sternum pain
5 spondylosis _____	e. malignant tumor of smooth muscle
6 patellectomy _____	f. abnormal condition of the backbone
7 sternodynia _____	g. pertaining to the ilium and femur
8 iliofemoral _____	h. abnormal growth of bone marrow cells
9 leiomysarcoma _____	i. incision into the skull
10 cephalomegaly _____	j. between the vertebrae

Practice 5.5 Define the following terms:

1. laminectomy _____
2. arthroplasty _____
3. chondroma _____
4. hypotonia _____
5. inositis _____
6. tenorrhaphy _____
7. pelvioscopy _____
8. atony _____

Table 5.4 Abbreviations Used for the Musculoskeletal System	
Abbreviation	**Meaning**
AE	above the elbow
AK	above the knee
ASF	anterior spinal fusion
BE	below the elbow
BK	below the knee
DJD	degenerative joint disease
DTR	deep tendon reflex
EMG	electromyography
Fx	fracture
IM	intramuscular
NSAIDs	nonsteriodal anti-inflammatory drugs
PT	physical therapy
ROM	range of motion
THA	total hip arthroplasty
TKA	total knee arthroplasty
TMJ	temporomandibular joint

3. The **cardiovascular system** consists of the heart, blood, and blood vessels. It transports oxygen and nutrients to the body tissues and helps the body to dispose of metabolic wastes. It is also called the circulatory system. The major components of this system are as follows:

   ■ **The heart**: It is a hollow muscular pumping organ that pumps the blood into the circulatory system through a network of arteries and veins by rhythmic contraction and dilation. Its size is about the size of the fist and it is located medial to the lungs along the body's midline in the thoracic region. The heart consists of four major chambers.

- The right atrium receives blood from the veins and pumps it to the right ventricle.
- The right ventricle receives blood from the right atrium and pumps it to the lungs, where it is loaded with oxygen.
- The left atrium receives oxygenated blood from the lungs and pumps it to the left ventricle.
- The left ventricle (the strongest chamber) pumps oxygen-rich blood to the rest of the body. The left ventricle's vigorous contractions create our blood pressure.
- **Blood vessels:** Blood vessels are the body's pathways that allow blood to flow quickly and efficiently from the heart to every region of the body and back again. The size of blood vessels corresponds with the amount of blood that passes through the vessel. All blood vessels contain a hollow area called the lumen through which blood is able to flow. Around the lumen is the wall of the vessel, which may be thin in the case of capillaries or very thick in the case of arteries. Blood vessels can be classified into three major types:
  - **Arteries**: An artery is a muscular vessel through which the oxygenated blood is conveyed from the heart to the various parts of the body. The small vessels that branch from arteries to transport the blood to the capillaries are called **arterioles**.
  - **Capillaries**: These are the smallest of blood vessels and distribute oxygenated blood from the arteries to the various body tissues. These also convey deoxygenated blood from the tissues to the veins.
  - **Veins:** They are blood vessels through which blood passes from the various parts of the body back to the heart. The small veins that collect blood from the capillaries and other tissues of the body back to the heart are referred to as **venules**.
- **Blood**: It is the red fluid or liquid that circulates through the heart, arteries, and veins and carries oxygen and nutrients to all body tissues (arterial blood). It also removes waste materials and carbon dioxide from the body tissues (venous blood). The blood consists of white and red cells, platelets, proteins, plasma (the liquid part of the blood that transports blood cells and other components through the body). The red cells (erythrocytes) contain hemoglobin that carries oxygen in the blood. The white blood cells (leukocytes) protect the body from infection and disease by killing the invading microbes. Finally, platelets are blood elements that help in clotting.

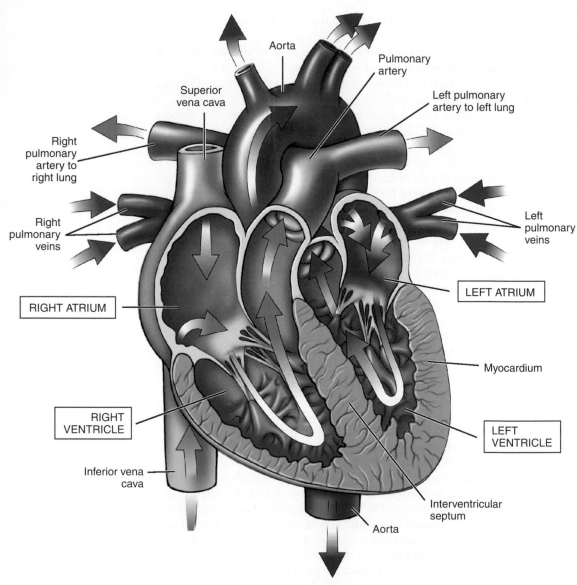

Aorta

Pulmonary artery

Superior vena cava

Left pulmonary artery to left lung

Right pulmonary artery to right lung

Left pulmonary veins

Right pulmonary veins

LEFT ATRIUM

RIGHT ATRIUM

Myocardium

RIGHT VENTRICLE

LEFT VENTRICLE

Inferior vena cava

Interventricular septum

Aorta

FIGURE 5.6 The components of the heart.

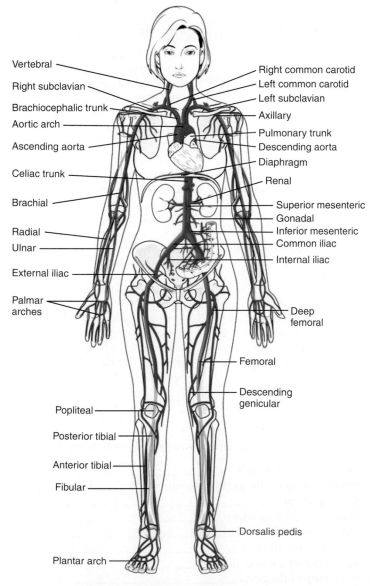

Vertebral

Right subclavian

Brachiocephalic trunk

Aortic arch

Ascending aorta

Celiac trunk

Brachial

Radial

Ulnar

External iliac

Palmar
arches

Popliteal

Posterior tibial

Anterior tibial

Fibular

Plantar arch

Right common carotid

Left common carotid

Left subclavian

Axillary

Pulmonary trunk

Descending aorta

Diaphragm

Renal

Superior mesenteric

Gonadal

Inferior mesenteric

Common iliac

Internal iliac

Deep
femoral

Femoral

Descending
genicular

Dorsalis pedis

FIGURE 5.7 Principal systemic arteries and veins.

Table 5.5 Roots for the Cardiovascular System

Root	Meaning	Example	Meaning
angi/o	vessels	angiogram	record of the blood vessels
aort/o	aorta	aortic	pertaining to the aorta
arteri/o	artery	arteriosclerosis	hardening of an artery
arteriol/o	arteriole	arteriolitis	inflammation of an arteriole
ather/o	fatty matter	atherosclerosis	hardening of the fatty substance
atri/o	atrium	interatrial	between the atria
cardi/o	heart	cardiology	study of the heart
coron/o	heart	coronary	pertaining to the artery
embol/o	plug	embolectomy	excision of an embolus
hemangi/o	blood vessels	hemangioma	abnormal mass of blood vessels
phleb/o	vein	phlebitis	inflammation of the vein
sept/o	septum	septostomy	opening of the septum to the outside of the body
sphygm/o	pulse	sphygmomanometer	instrument for measuring blood pressure
thromb/o	blood clot	thrombocytosis	abnormal increase in blood platelets in the blood
valv/o	valve	valvar	▪ pertaining to the valve
valvul/o		valvuloplasty	▪ plastic repair of a valve
vas/o	vessel	vasodepressor	agent that lowers blood pressure
vascul/o	vessel	cardiovascular	pertaining to the heart and vessels
ven/o	vein	intravenous	within the vein
ventricul/o	cavity	supraventricular	above the ventricular
venul/o	venule	venulitis	inflammation of the venule

Practice 5.6 Write the medical term for each of the following definitions.

1. disease of heart muscle _____
2. inflammation of the membrane surrounding the heart _____
3. X-ray of a vein _____
4. plastic repair of an artery _____
5. inflammation of a vein _____
6. rupture of the heart _____
7. separation of a blood clot _____
8. hardening of the aorta _____
9. removal of an embolus _____
10. poisonous to the heart _____

Practice 5.7 Use the root **angi/o** to write words with the following meanings:

1. any disease of a vessel _____
2. dilation of a vessel _____

3. plastic repair of a vessel _____
4. formation of a vessel _____
5. softening of a vessel _____
6. record of a vessel _____

Table 5.6 Abbreviations Used for the Cardiovascular System	
Abbreviation	**Meaning**
ACS	acute coronary syndrome
AED	automated external defibrillator
AF	atrial fibrillation
AMI	acute myocardial infarction
AR	aortic regurgitation
AS	aortic stenosis
ASD	atrial septal defect
ASHD	arteriosclerosis heart disease
AST	angiotension sensitivity test
AV	arteriovenous
BP	blood pressure
BPM	beats per minute
CABG	coronary artery bypass grafting
CAD	coronary artery disease
CCU	coronary care unit
CHF	congestive heart failure
CO	cardiac output
CPR	cardiopulmonary resuscitation
CVA	cerebrovascular accident
DVT	deep venous thrombosis
ECG	electrocardiogram
ECHO	echocardiogram
ETT	exercise tolerance test
HDL	high-density lipoprotein
HF	heart failure
HTN	hypertension
LDL	low-density lipoprotein
LV	left ventricle
LVH	left ventricular hypertrophy
MI	myocardial infarction
MR	mitral regurgitation
MVP	mitral valve prolapse
NSR	normal sinus rhythm
PCI	percutaneous coronary intervention
SV	stroke volume
VT	ventricular tachycardia

4. The **lymphatic (lymph) system** works in close cooperation with the circulatory system. It consists of the lymph, lymphatic vessels, spleen, tonsils, adenoids, and thymus. It is a network of tissues and organs that helps the body to get rid of toxins and waste materials. Its major role is to transport a fluid, called the lymph, that contains leukocytes throughout the body in order to fight infection. The lymphatic system consists of hundreds of nodes distributed in different locations in the human body. The major functions of the lymphatic system include:

- It is part of the immune system.
- It maintains fluid balance.
- It helps in absorbing fats and fat-soluble nutrients.
- The lymph nodes swell in response to infection.
- The lymph nodes filter lymph and provide part of the adaptive immune response to new pathogens.

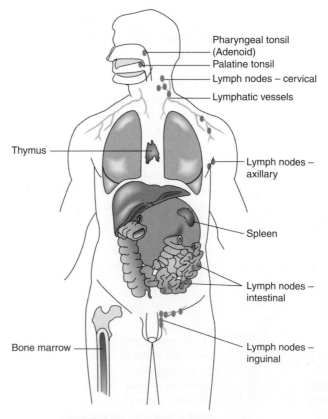

FIGURE 5.8 The lymph and immune system.

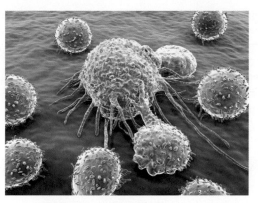

FIGURE 5.9 Lymphocytes attack a cancer cell.

Table 5.7 Roots for the Lymphatic System

Root	Meaning	Example	Meaning
aden/o	gland	adenoid	resembling a gland
lymph/o	lymph	lymphocyte	white blood cells associated with the immune response
lymphaden/o	lymph nodes	lymphadenopathy	disease affecting the lymph nodes
lymphangi/o	lymphatic vessels	lymphangitis	inflammation of the lymphatic vessels
splen/o	spleen	splenomegaly	enlargement of the spleen
thym/o	thymus	thymectomy	excision of the thymus
tonsill/o	tonsil	tonsillar	pertaining to a tonsil

Practice 5.8 Use the appropriate root to produce words with the following meanings.

1. inflammation of the lymphatic vessels _____
2. a tumor of lymphatic tissue _____
3. excision of the lymph nodes _____
4. pertaining to the thymus gland _____
5. inflammation of a tonsil _____
6. pain in the spleen _____
7. X-ray study of the lymphatic vessels _____

Practice 5.9 Write the adjective form of the following words:

1. atrium _____
2. thymus _____
3. vein _____
4. septum _____
5. spleen _____

Table 5.8 Abbreviations Used for the Lymphatic System	
Abbreviation	**Meaning**
AIDS	acquired immunodeficiency syndrome
ALL	acute lymphocytic leukemia
CLL	chronic lymphocytic leukemia
CML	chronic myelogenous leukemia
ELISA	enzyme-linked immunosorbent assay
HAART	highly active antiretroviral therapy
HD	Hodgkin disease
HIV	human immunodeficiency virus
IgA, D, E, G	immunoglobulin A, D, E, G
MAC	mycobacterium avium complex
PCP	pneumocystic pneumonia
SLE	systemic lupus erythematosus

5. The **nervous system** consists of the brain, spinal cord, nerves, and sense organs, such as the eye and the ear, and all the nerves that connect these organs with the body. It is responsible for the control and communication among its various parts. The nervous system comprises a complicated number of nerves and specialized cells called neurons. These are nerve cells whose function is to receive signals from sensory cells and from other neurons and send signals to muscle neurons as well as other neurons.

The nervous system comprises two major components: the central nervous system (CNS) and the peripheral nervous system (PNS). The CNS consists of the brain and the spinal cord, whereas the PNS consists of the nerves outside the brain and the spinal cord. The peripheral nerves connect the CNS to sensory organs including the eyes and ears as well as to other parts of the body such as the muscles, blood vessels, and glands.

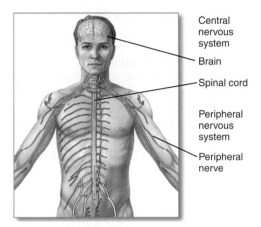

Central
nervous
system

Brain

Spinal cord

Peripheral
nervous
system

Peripheral
nerve

FIGURE 5.10 The peripheral nervous system.

The following is a description of the major components of the nervous system and their functions.

1. **The brain** is the part of the CNS that is enclosed in the skull. It consists of two halves: the left hemisphere and the right hemisphere; each of which has its own functions. The brain is the controller of the body because it is the primary receiver, organizer, and distributor of information for the entire human body.

   The brain consists of the following major parts:

   - **The cerebrum** is the largest part of the brain and it is responsible for most of the functions of the brain. It consists of four sections called lobes: the temporal lobe, the occipital lobe, the parietal lobe, and the frontal lobe. It is also divided into the right and left hemispheres that are connected with each other by axons whose function is to convey messages from one hemisphere to another.

   - **The cerebellum** is often referred to as the "little brain." It is located behind the top part of the brain stem where the spinal cord is connected with the brain. It receives information from the sensory systems, the spinal cord, and other parts of the brain. It is also responsible for regulating motor movements.

   - **The brain stem** is the part of the brain that is connected to the spinal cord. It controls the flow of messages between the brain and the remaining parts of the body. It also controls the basic functions of the body such as heartbeat, blood pressure, swallowing, and breathing. It is composed of the midbrain, pons, and medulla oblongata. The limbic system is part of the brain stem that consists of glands which play an important role in emotions and the formation of memories. It includes the amygdala, hippocampus, hypothalamus, and thalamus. The limbic system is responsible for three major functions: emotions, memories, and arousal (or stimulation).

2. **Spinal cord** is the column of nerve tissue that is connected to the brain and lies within the vertebral canal and from which the spinal nerves emerge. It extends from the medulla oblongata in the brain stem to the lumbar region of the vertebral column. Thirty-one pairs of spinal nerves originate in the spinal cord: 8 cervical, 12 thoracic, 5 lumbar, 5 sacral, and 1 coccygeal. The spinal cord and the brain constitute the CNS.

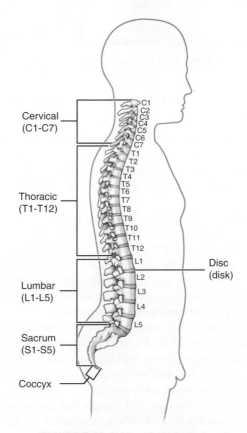

FIGURE 5.11 Division of spinal column.

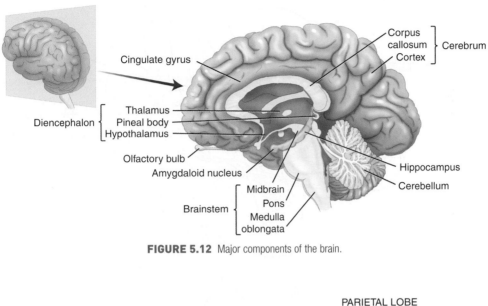

FIGURE 5.12 Major components of the brain.

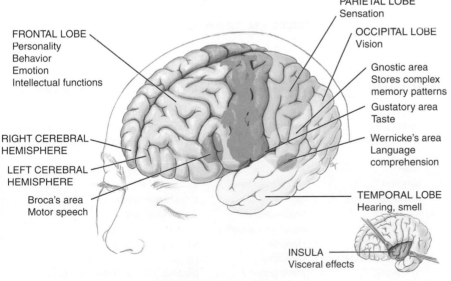

FIGURE 5.13 Lobes of the brain.

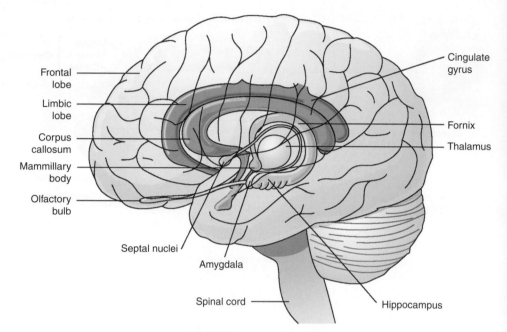

FIGURE 5.14 The limbic system.

Table 5.9 Roots for the Nervous System

Root	Meaning	Example	Meaning
cerebell/o	cerebellum	supracerebellar	above the cerebellum
cerebr/o	cerebrum	cerebral	pertaining to the largest part of the brain
cortic/o	cerebral cortex	corticospinal	pertaining to the cerebral cortex and spinal cord
encephal/o	brain	encephalitis	inflammation of the brain
gangli/o, ganglion/o	ganglion	ganglionectomy	excision of the ganglion
gli/o	neuroglia	glioma	a neuroglial tumor
kinesi/o	movement	bradykinesia	slow movement
lept/o	thin, slender	leptomeningopathy	disease of meninges
lex/o	word, phrase	dyslexia	difficulty in reading
medull/o	medulla oblongata	medullary	pertaining to the medulla
mening/o, meninge/o	meninges	meningococci	bacteria that infect the meninges
myel/o	spinal cord	myelitis	inflammation of the spinal cord
narc/o	stupor	narcosis	state of stupor
neur/o	nerve	neuroplasty	plastic repair of the nerve
psych/o	mind	psychoactive	acting on the mind
radicul/o	spinal nerve root	radiculitis	inflammation of the spinal nerve root
somn/o, somn/i	sleep	somnolence	sleepiness
thalam/o	thalamus	thalamotomy	incision into the thalamus
ventricul/o	cavity	intraventricular	within a ventricle

Practice 5.10 Match each of the following terms in column A with its meaning in column B.

A	B
1 myeloplegia _____	a. tumor of a ganglion
2 dyskinesia _____	b. within the cerebellum
3 neurotripsy _____	c. lack of sleep
4 encephalography _____	d. paralysis of the spinal cord
5 craniometer _____	e. radiography of the brain
6 ganglioma _____	f. outside the cerebrum
7 neuropathy _____	g. crushing of a nerve
8 insomnia _____	h. instrument for measuring the skull
9 intracerebellar _____	i. difficult movement
10 extracerebral _____	j. any disease of the nerve

Practice 5.11 Complete the following sentences with the proper word.

1. Destruction of nerve is called _____.
2. Any disease of the spinal nerve root is also termed _____.
3. The term psychogenic means originating in the _____.
4. Outside the medulla is called _____.
5. Radiograph of a ventricle is called _____.

Table 5.10 Abbreviations Used for the Nervous System	
Abbreviation	**Meaning**
AD	Alzheimer disease
CNS	central nervous system
CSF	cerebrospinal fluid
CVA	cerebrovascular accident
EEG	electroencephalogram
LP	lumbar puncture
MS	multiple sclerosis
TENS	transcutaneous electrical nerve stimulation
TIA	transient ischemic attack
ALS	amyotrophic lateral sclerosis
PNS	peripheral nervous system
BBB	blood–brain barrier
CT	computed tomography
ADHD	attention deficit hyperactivity disorder
ANS	autonomic nervous system
ICP	intracranial pressure
MRI	magnetic resonance imaging
MRA	magnetic resonance angiogram

6. The **endocrine system** includes all hormone-producing glands and cells such as the pituitary gland, thyroid gland, pancreas, parathyroid glands, adrenal glands, pancreas, ovaries (in females), and testicles (in males). Its major function is to regulate body functions pertaining to metabolism, growth and development, tissue function, sexual function, reproduction, sleep and mood by means of hormones.

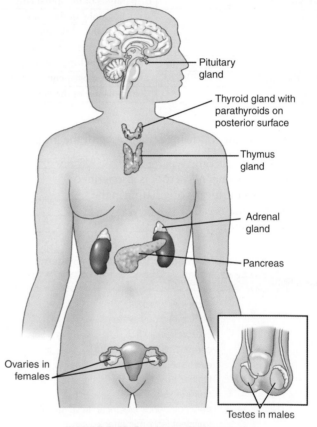

Pituitary gland

Thyroid gland with parathyroids on posterior surface

Thymus gland

Adrenal gland

Pancreas

Ovaries in females

Testes in males

FIGURE 5.15 Female reproductive system.

Table 5.11 Roots for the Endocrine System

Root	Meaning	Example	Meaning
aden/o	gland	adenopathy	lymph node disease
adren/o, adrenal/o	adrenal glands	adrenomegaly	enlargement of the adrenal glands
adrenocortic/o	adrenal cortex	adrenocorticotropic	acting on the adrenal cortex
gluc/o	glucose	glucogenesis	production of glucose
glyc/o	glycogen	glycolysis	conversion of glycogen to glucose
gonad/o	sex glands	gonadotropin	hormone that aids in the growth of gonads
hypophys/o	pituitary gland	hypophyseal	pertaining to the pituitary gland
insul/o	pancreatic islets	insular	pertaining to the islet cells
oophor/o	ovary	oophorectomy	excision of the ovary
orch/o	testis	orchitis	■ inflammation of the testis
orchi/o		orchiopexy	■ fixation of the testis
orchid/o		orchidectomy	■ excision of the testis
ovary/o	ovary	ovarian cyst	a small fluid-filled sac that develops in a woman's ovaries
pancreat/o	pancreas	pancreatitis	inflammation of the pancreas
parathyroid/o	parathyroid	parathyroidectomy	excision of the parathyroid glands
thyr/o, thyroid/o	thyroid gland	thyrotoxic	having excessive amounts of thyroid hormones
thyroaden/o	thyroid gland	thyroadenitis	inflammation of the thyroid gland

Practice 5.12 Write the name of each numbered part in the table below.

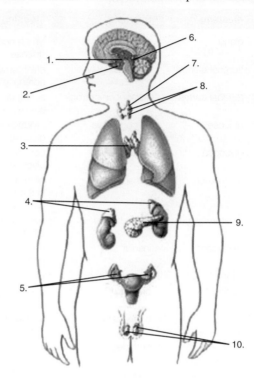

	Name
1	
2	
3	
4	
5	
6	
7	
8	
9	
10	

Practice 5.13 Use **glyc/o** to build words that mean:

1. blood condition of excessive glucose _____
2. blood condition of deficiency of glucose _____
3. formation of glycogen _____

Practice 5.14 Supply the missing part of the term.

1. removal of a gland is…….........ectomy
2. removal of the pituitary gland is……………ectomy
3. removal of an adrenal gland is……………ectomy
4. removal of the thymus gland is……………ectomy
5. removal of part of the pancreas is……..........ectomy
6. removal of the thyroid gland is……..........ectomy
7. removal of one or more of the thyroid gland is……..........ectomy

Table 5.12 Abbreviations Used for the Endocrine System	
Abbreviation	**Meaning**
A1c	glycated hemoglobin
ACTH	adrenocorticotropic hormone
ADH	antidiuretic hormone
BMI	body mass index
BMR	basal metabolic rate
DI	diabetes ketoacidosis
DM	diabetes mellitus
FSH	follicle-stimulating hormone
FTI	free thyroxine index
GH	growth hormone
GTT	glucose tolerance test
HbA1c	hemoglobin A1c measures the average amount of glucose in red blood cells
HCG	human chorionic gonadotropin
HRT	hormone replacement therapy
IFG	impaired fasting blood glucose
K^+	potassium
LH	luteinizing hormone
MEN	multiple endocrine neoplasia
Na^+	sodium
OGTT	oral glucose tolerance test
PGH	pituitary growth hormone

Continued

Table 5.12 Abbreviations Used for the Endocrine System—Cont'd	
Abbreviation	**Meaning**
PRL	prolactin
PTH	parathyroid hormone
RAI	radioactive iodine
STH	somatotropin hormone
T3	triiodothyronine
T4	thyroxine
TBG	thyroxine-binding globulin
TFT	thyroid function test
TSH	thyroid-stimulating hormone

7. The **respiratory system** includes the nose, pharynx, larynx, trachea, bronchi, and lungs.

It transports air into and out of the lungs. It facilitates the diffusion of the oxygen into the blood stream and receives carbon dioxide from the blood and exhales it. The respiratory system performs a number of functions. It facilitates the exchange of gases between the air and the blood through breathing, inhalation, and exhalation. The following are the major functions of this system:

1. Breathing through inhalation and exhalation: In this process, air is inhaled through the nasal and oral cavities down to the pharynx, larynx, and trachea into the lungs. The air is then exhaled and flows back through the same channel.
2. Exchanging gases between the lungs and the blood (external respiration): In this process, oxygen is exchanged for carbon dioxide through a huge number of microscopic sacs called alveoli.
3. Exchanging gases between the blood and the body tissues (internal respiration): In this process, oxygen is delivered to the body tissues through the bloodstream and carbon dioxide is removed through internal respiration.
4. Creating sound: When the air is exhaled from the lungs through the trachea into the larynx, it causes the vocal cords to vibrate and produce sounds.
5. Smelling (olfaction): The chemical process starts in the nasal cavity as air passes through the nose.

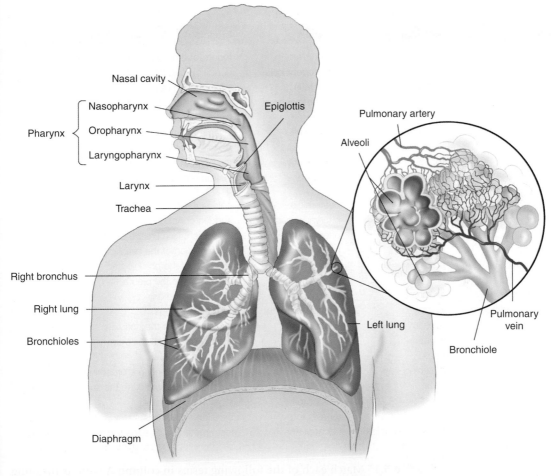

FIGURE 5.16 The respiratory system.

Table 5.13 Roots for the Respiratory System

Root	Meaning	Example	Meaning
adenoid/o	adenoid	adenoidectomy	excision of the adenoid
alveol/o	alveolus	alveolitis	inflammation of the alveoli
anthrac/o	coal dust	anthracosis	abnormal condition of the coal dust
bronch/o, bronchi/o	bronchus	bronchitis	inflammation of the lining of the bronchial tubes
bronchiol/o	bronchiole	bronchiolectasis	dilatation of the bronchioles

Continued

Table 5.13 Roots for the Respiratory System—Cont'd

Root	Meaning	Example	Meaning
capn/o	carbon dioxide	capnogram	record of the carbon dioxide in expired air
coni/o	dust	pneumoconiosis	condition of dust in the lung
epiglott/o	epiglottis	epiglottitis	inflammation of the epiglottis
laryng/o	larynx (voice box)	laryngoscope	instrument to visually examine the larynx
lob/o	lobe of the lung	lobectomy	excision of the lobe
mediastin/o	mediastinum	mediastinitis	inflammation of the mediastinum
nas/o	nose	nasal	pertaining to the nose
or/o	mouth	oropharynx	the part of the mouth that lies behind the mouth
ox/o	oxygen	oximeter	instrument to measure oxygen saturation of blood
pector/o	chest	pectoralgia	pain in the chest
pharyng/o	throat	pharyngospasm	sudden contraction of the throat
phon/o	voice	phonometer	instrument to measure sounds
phren/o	diaphragm	phrenitis	inflammation of the diaphragm
phrenic/o	phrenic nerve	phrenicotripsy	crushing of the phrenic nerve
pleur/o	pleura	pleurocentesis	puncture into the pleura
pneumon/o	air, lung	pneumonia	lung inflammation
pulm/o, pulmon/o	lungs	extrapulmonary	outside the lungs
rhin/o	nose	rhinoplasty	plastic repair of the nose
sept/o	septum	septoplasty	plastic repair of the septum
sinus/o	sinus	sinusotomy	incision of a sinus
spir/o	breathing	spirometer	instrument to measure breathing
steth/o	chest	stethoscope	instrument for listening to the sound of the chest
thorac/o	chest	thoracotomy	incision of the chest
tonsil/o	tonsil	tonsillectomy	excision of the tonsils
trache/o	trachea (windpipe)	tracheotome	instrument to incise the trachea

Practice 5.15 Match each of the following terms in column A with its meaning in column B.

A	B
1 alveolar _____	a. throat
2 phrenic _____	b. voice box
3 larynx _____	c. windpipe
4 trachea _____	d. thin-walled sac through which gases can pass into and out of the bloodstream
5 epiglottis _____	e. lymph tissue in the throat
6 bronchiole _____	f. small bronchial tube
7 air sac _____	g. one of two tubes that carry air from the windpipe to the lungs
8 pharynx _____	h. flap of cartilage over the mouth of the trachea
9 bronchial tube _____	i. pertaining to the diaphragm
10 tonsils _____	j. pertaining to an air sac

Practice 5.16 Write the medical term for each of the following definitions:

1. within the pleura _____
2. above the diaphragm _____
3. any disease of the lungs _____
4. surgical incision of the phrenic nerve _____
5. record of breathing volume _____
6. pertaining to the bronchioles _____

Table 5.14 Abbreviations Used for the Respiratory System

Abbreviation	Meaning
A&P	auscultation and percussion
ABG	arterial blood gas
AFB	acid-fast bacillus
ARDS	acute respiratory distress syndrome
ARF	acute respiratory failure
BS	breath sounds
C	compliance
CF	cystic fibrosis
CO_2	carbon dioxide
COLD	chronic obstructive lung disease
COPD	chronic obstructive pulmonary disease
CPAP	continuous positive airway pressure
CPR	cardiopulmonary resuscitation
CXR	chest radiograph
DOE	dyspnea on exertion
FRC	functional residual capacity
FVC	forced vital capacity
HPS	hantavirus pulmonary syndrome
IC	inspiratory capacity
IPPB	intermittent positive pressure breathing
IPPV	intermittent positive pressure ventilation
IRV	inspiratory reserve volume
LLL	left lower lobe
LUL	left upper lobe
MBC	maximal breathing capacity
MDI	metered dose inhaler
PE	pulmonary embolism
PEEP	positive end expiratory pressure
PFT	pulmonary function test
R	respiration
RDS	respiratory distress syndrome
RLL	right lower lobe
RML	right middle lobe
RUL	right upper lobe

Continued

Table 5.14 Abbreviations Used for the Respiratory System—Cont'd

Abbreviation	Meaning
RV	residual volume
SARS	severe acute respiratory syndrome
SIDS	sudden infant death syndrome
SOB	shortness of breath
SpO_2	oxygen percent saturation
TGV	thoracic gas volume
TLC	total lung capacity
TPR	temperature, pulse, and respiration
URI	upper respiratory infection
VATS	video-assisted thoracic surgery
VC	vital capacity
VP	ventilation-perfusion

8. The **digestive system** is responsible for getting food into and out of the body in order to keep it healthy. It starts at the oral cavity including the teeth, the tongue, salivary glands, pharynx, esophagus, stomach, the liver, gallbladder, pancreas, small intestines, large intestines, and ends with the anus. This long tract is called the alimentary canal or the gastrointestinal (GI) tract. This system breaks down and absorbs food for use by cells and eliminates solid and other waste materials.

Digestion is a complex process in which food is turned into nutrients that the body uses for energy and growth. The digestive system consists of a number of body parts that work together in order to coordinate the movement of food through the alimentary canal and produce enzymes and hormones necessary to breakdown the food. The following is a brief description of the body organs involved in the digestive system.

- **Mouth**: The oral cavity includes the tongue, the teeth, and the salivary glands. Digestion starts in the mouth when the food is chewed and broken down into an easily digested form.
- **Esophagus**: It is the tube that connects the pharynx (throat) to the stomach. It receives the food from the mouth and passes it to the stomach.
- **Stomach**: It is a muscular organ located in the upper abdomen under the ribs. It receives food from the esophagus and passes it to the small intestine. The stomach secretes acids and enzymes in order to digest food.
- **Small intestine**: It is the part of the body that directly receives the food from the stomach. It is about 5-m long and is narrower than the large intestine. It consists of three parts: the duodenum, jejunum, and ileum.

- **Pancreas**: Its major function is to secrete digestive enzymes into the duodenum in order to break down protein, fats, and carbohydrates. The pancreas also secretes insulin that metabolizes sugar in the blood.
- **Liver**: The major function of the liver is to process the nutrients absorbed from the small intestine. It secretes bile that is necessary for digesting fat.
- **Gallbladder**: It is a small sac-shaped organ beneath the liver where bile secreted by the liver is stored. It releases this bile into the duodenum to facilitate the absorption and digestion of fats.
- **Colon**: It is also called the large intestine. It is connected to the small intestine at the ileum (last part of the small intestine). It consists of the ascending colon, the transverse colon, the descending colon, and the sigmoid colon.
- **Rectum**: It is the final part of the large intestine that connects it to the anus.
- **Anus**: It is the last part of the alimentary canal through which stool passes out.

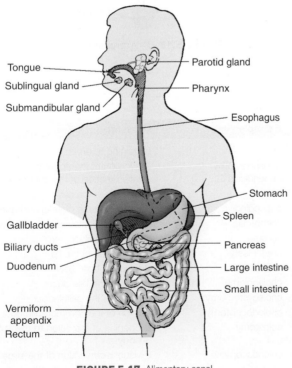

FIGURE 5.17 Alimentary canal.

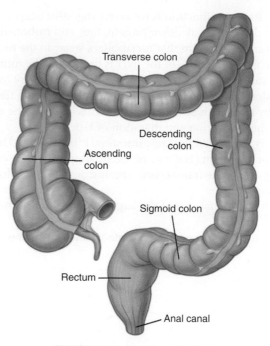

FIGURE 5.18 Colon (large intestine).

Table 5.15 Roots for the Digestive System

Root	Meaning	Example	Meaning
an/o	anus	anal	pertaining to anus
append/o appendic/o	appendix	appendectomy appendicitis	▪ excision of the appendix ▪ inflammation of the appendix
bil/o	bile	biliary	pertaining to the bile
bucc/o	cheek	buccogingival	pertaining to the cheeks and gums
cec/o	cecum	cecoptosis	downward displacement of the cecum
celi/o	abdomen	celioma	tumor of the abdomen
cheil/o	lip	cheiloplasty	plastic repair of the lip
chol/o, chol/e	bile, gall	cholestasis	stoppage of bile flow
cholangi/o	bile duct	cholangioma	cancer of the bile ducts
cholecyst/o	gallbladder	cholecystectomy	excision of the gallbladder
choledoch/o	common bile duct	choledochotomy	incision of the common bile duct
col/o	large intestine	colostomy	▪ opening of the colon to the outside of the body
colon/o		colonoscopy	▪ visual examination of the large intestine

Table 5.15 Roots for the Digestive System—Cont'd

Root	Meaning	Example	Meaning
dent/o, dent/i	tooth	edentulous	without/lacking teeth
duoden/o	duodenum	duodenostomy	opening of the duodenum to the outside of the body
enter/o	small intestine	dysentery	infectious disease of the intestine
esophagi/o	esophagus	esophageal	pertaining to the esophagus
gastr/o	stomach	gastroscopy	visual examination of the stomach
gingiv/o	gum	gingivitis	inflammation of the gum
gloss/o	tongue	glossoplegia	paralysis of the tongue
gnath/o	jaw	prognathic	pertaining to the jaw
hepat/o	liver	hepatitis	inflammation of the liver
ile/o	ileum	ileitis	inflammation of the ileum
jejun/o	jejunum	gastrojejunostomy	communication between the stomach and jejunum
labi/o	lip	labium	lip structure
lingu/o	tongue	lingual	pertaining to the tongue
odont/o	tooth	orthodontics	treatment of irregularities in teeth and jaws
or/o	mouth	oral	pertaining to the mouth
palat/o	palate	palatine	pertaining to the palate
pancreat/o	pancreas	pancreatitis	inflammation of the pancreas
peritone/o	peritoneum	peritonitis	inflammation of the peritoneum
proct/o	rectum	proctopexy	fixation of the rectum
pylor/o	pylorus	pyloroplasty	plastic repair of the pylorus
rect/o	rectum	rectocele	hernia of the rectum
sial/o	saliva	sialogram	record of the salivary gland
sialaden/o	salivary gland	sialoadenitis	inflammation of the salivary glands
sigmoid/o	sigmoid colon	sigmoidoscopy	visual examination of the sigmoid colon
steat/o	fats	steatorrhea	greater than normal amounts of fats in the feces
stomat/o	mouth	xerostomia	dryness of the mouth
uvul/o	uvula	uvulotome	instrument for incising the uvula

Practice 5.17 Write the proper term for each of the following definitions:

1. excision of gums _____
2. partial or complete excision of the tongue _____
3. repair of the esophagus _____
4. removal of the stomach _____
5. communication between the stomach and jejunum _____
6. surgical repair of the small intestine _____
7. suture of the bile duct _____
8. removal of the gallbladder _____
9. surgical repair of the rectum _____
10. inflammation of the pancreas _____

Practice 5.18 Label each numbered part. Write its name in the table below.

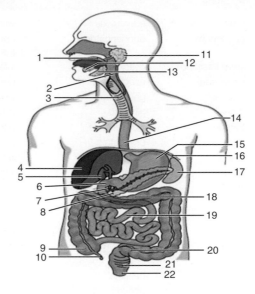

esophagus	pharynx	trachea	pancreas	sigmoid colon	small intestine	
common bile duct	liver	gallbladder	cecum	appendix	rectum	stomach
diaphragm	anus	duodenum	mouth	parotid	sublingual	subman-dibular
large intestine	spleen					

	Name
1	
2	
3	
4	
5	
6	
7	
8	
9	
10	
11	

	Name
12	
13	
14	
15	
16	
17	
18	
19	
20	
21	
22	

Table 5.16 Abbreviations Used for the Digestive System

Abbreviation	Meaning
ALT	alanine transaminase
AST	aspartate transaminase
BE	barium enema
BM	bowel movement
BMI	body mass index
EGD	esophagogastroduodenoscopy
ERCP	endoscopic retrograde cholangiopancreatography
FAP	familial adenomatous polyposis
GB	gallbladder
GERD	gastroesophageal reflux disease
GI	gastrointestinal
HAV	hepatitis A virus
HCl	hydrochloric acid
IBD	inflammatory bowel disease
IBS	irritable bowel syndrome
LES	lower esophageal sphincter
LFTs	liver function tests
NPO	nothing through mouth
PPI	proton pump inhibitor
TPN	total parenteral nutrition
UGI	upper gastrointestinal

9. **The urinary system** is known as the renal system or the excretory system. It is a group of organs that work together in order to filter out excess fluids and other substances from the blood in the form of urine that is produced by the kidneys and collected in the urinary bladder and then excreted through the urethra. The major function of this system is to remove liquid waste from the blood in the form of urine and to keep a stable balance of salts and other substances in the blood. Therefore, this system is the drainage system of the body. It consists of the kidneys, ureters, bladder, and urethra.

Kidneys: These are two bean-shaped organs located just below the rib cage, one on each side of the spine in the abdominal region. The major function of the kidneys is to filter the blood from waste products, chemicals, and unneeded water. Urine collects in the renal pelvis in the middle of each kidney, then it drains through the ureter to the bladder where it is stored until it is eliminated.

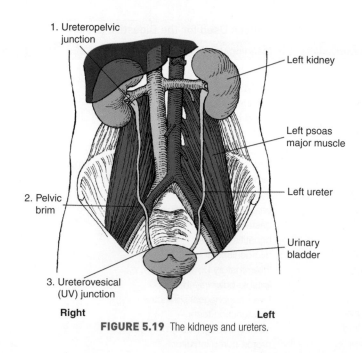

FIGURE 5.19 The kidneys and ureters.

Ureters: These are muscular tubes through which the urine passes from the kidneys to the bladder.

Bladder: It is a muscular sac in the pelvis above and behind the pubic bone. It stores the urine that it receives from the kidneys and empties it voluntarily through the urethra that is located at the bottom of the bladder.

Urethra: It is the tube that carries the urine from the bladder to the outside of the body.

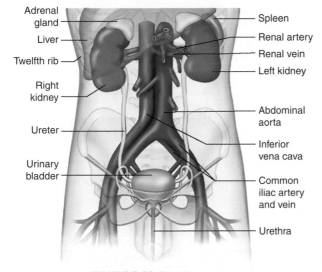

FIGURE 5.20 The urinary system.

Table 5.17 Roots for the Urinary System

Root	Meaning	Example	Meaning
cali/o	calyx	calioplasty	▪ plastic repair of the calyx
calic/o		calicectomy	▪ excision of the calyx
cyst/o	urinary bladder	cystitis	inflammation of the urinary bladder
glomerul/o	glomerulus	glomerulitis	inflammation of the glomerulus
lith/o	stone	lithotripsy	crushing of a stone
meat/o	meatus	meatotomy	incision of the meatus
nephr/o	kidney	nephrologist	specialist in the study and treatment of kidney diseases
pyel/o	renal pelvis	pyelogram	record of the renal pelvis
ren/o	kidney	renal	pertaining to the kidney
trigon/o	trigone	trigonitis	inflammation of the trigone
ur/o	urine	uremia	▪ having urea in the blood
urin/o		nocturia	▪ urination during the night
ureter/o	ureter	ureterectasis	dilation of the ureter
urethra/o	urethra	urethrostenosis	narrowing of the urethra
vesic/o	urinary bladder	vesical	pertaining to the urinary bladder

Practice 5.19 Use the root **nephr/o** to produce a medical term for each of the following definitions:

1. surgical removal of the kidney _____
2. study of the kidney _____
3. softening of the kidney _____
4. substances that are harmful to the kidney _____
5. any disease of the kidney _____
6. specialist in the study and treatment of the kidney _____
7. imaging of the kidney _____
8. incision to remove a kidney stone _____
9. inflammation of the renal pelvis and other kidney parts _____
10. tumor in the kidney _____

Practice 5.20 Match each of the following terms in column A with its meaning in column B.

A	B
1 ureterectomy _____	a. abnormal condition of kidney stone
2 intravesical _____	b. having blood in the urine
3 renal pelvis _____	c. visual examination of the urinary bladder
4 urinary bladder _____	d. excision of a ureter
5 urethra _____	e. tube that leads from the bladder to the outside of the body
6 ureter _____	f. one of two tubes that passes urine from the kidney to the urinary bladder
7 kidney _____	g. muscular sac that holds urine
8 cystoscopy _____	h. organ behind the abdomen that makes urine by filtering waste from the blood
9 nephrolithiasis _____	i. central section of the kidney
10 hematuria _____	j. within the urinary bladder

Table 5.18 Abbreviations Used for the Urinary System.

Abbreviation	Meaning
A/G	albumin/globulin
ADH	antidiuretic hormone
AGN	acute glomerulonephritis
ARF	acute renal failure
BNO	bladder neck obstruction
BUN	blood urea nitrogen
CAPD	continuous ambulatory peritoneal dialysis
Cath	catheter
CCPD	continuous cyclic peritoneal dialysis
CFR	glomerular filtration rate
CKD	chronic kidney disease
CRF	chronic renal failure
DRE	digital rectal examination
ESRD	end-stage renal disease
ESWL	extracorporeal shock wave lithotripsy
HD	hemodialysis
IVP	intravenous pyelogram/pyelography
IVU	intravenous urography
KUB	kidney, ureter, bladder (radiography)
PKU	phenylketonuria
RP	retrograde pyelogram
SG	specific gravity
UA	urinalysis
UTI	urinary tract infection
VCUG	voiding cystourethrogram

10. The **reproductive system:** Males and females have their own reproductive systems that serve different functions. The male reproductive system consists of the testes, prostate glands, sperm ducts, urethra, and penis. The female reproductive system consists of the vagina, uterus, ovaries, and fallopian tubes. Each system has its own functions that serve the general reproduction function in both males and females. The male reproductive system performs the following major functions:

   - producing, maintaining, and transporting sperm and protective fluid (semen)
   - discharging sperm into the female reproductive tract during sex
   - producing and secreting male sex hormones necessary for maintaining the male reproductive system

Most of the organs of the male reproductive system are located outside the body.

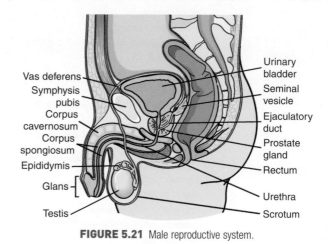

Vas deferens
Symphysis pubis
Corpus cavernosum
Corpus spongiosum
Epididymis
Glans
Testis

Urinary bladder
Seminal vesicle
Ejaculatory duct
Prostate gland
Rectum
Urethra
Scrotum

FIGURE 5.21 Male reproductive system.

The female reproductive system performs the following functions:

- producing female egg cells essential for reproduction; they are called ova or oocytes
- protecting and nourishing the embryo until birth
- producing female sex hormones that maintain the reproductive cycle

The female reproductive system includes organs inside and outside the body.

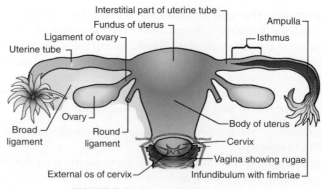

Interstitial part of uterine tube
Fundus of uterus
Ligament of ovary
Uterine tube
Ampulla
Isthmus

Ovary
Broad ligament
Round ligament
Body of uterus
Cervix
Vagina showing rugae
External os of cervix
Infundibulum with fimbriae

FIGURE 5.22 Female reproductive system.

Table 5.19 Roots for the Male and Female Reproductive Systems

Root	Meaning	Example	Meaning
amni/o	amnion	amniocentesis	test of amniotic fluid by insertion of a needle into the amnion
balan/o	penis	balanitis	inflammation of the penis
cervic/o	cervix	cervicitis	inflammation of the cervix
clitor/o	clitoris	clitorectomy	excision of the clitoris
colp/o	vagina	colpostenosis	narrowing of the vagina
embry/o	embry/o	embryonic	pertaining to the embryo
epididym/o	epididymis	epididymotomy	incision into the epididymis
episi/o	vulva	episiotomy	incision into the perineum
fet/o	fetus	fetometry	measurement of a fetus
galact/o	milk	galactopoiesis	milk production
gynec/o, gyn/o	female	gynecologist	specialist in the study and treatment of women's diseases
hyster/o	uterus	hysterectomy	excision of the uterus
lact/o	milk	lactogenesis	milk production
mamm/o	breast	mammography	imaging of the breast
mast/o	breast	mastitis	inflammation of the breast
men/o	menstruation	menopause	stoppage of the menstruation
metr/o metri/o	uterus	metropathy endometrium	■ disease of the uterus ■ within the uterus
nat/o	birth	prenatal	pertaining to before birth
o/o	egg	oocyte	egg cells
oophor/o	ovary	oophoritis	inflammation of the ovary
orch/o, orchi/o, orchid/o	testis	orchitis orchiopexy orchidectomy	■ inflammation of the testis ■ fixation of the testis ■ excision of the testis
osche/o	scrotum	oscheal	pertaining to scrotum
ov/i ov/o	egg	ovoid	egg-shaped
ovari/o	ovary	ovariopexy	surgical fixation of the ovary
ovul/o	ovum, egg cells	ovulatory	pertaining to ovulation
perine/o	perineum	perinecele	hernia in the perineum
prostat/o	prostate	prostatometer	instrument for measuring the prostate
salping/o	fallopian tube	salpingitis	inflammation of the fallopian tubes
sperm/i, spermat/o	semen	polyspermia	secretion of excess semen
test/o	testis, testicle	testosterone	hormone produced in the testis
toc/o	labor	dystocia	difficult labor
uter/o	uterus	uteroplastsy	surgical repair of the uterus
vagin/o	vagina	vaginitis	inflammation of the vagina
varic/o	dilated vein	varicocele	swelling of a dilated vein
vas/o	vas deferens	vasostomy	opening of the ductus deferens
vesicul/o	seminal vesicle	vesiculogram	radiograph of a seminal vesicle
vulv/o	vulva	vulvitis	inflammation of the vulva

Practice 5.21 Define the following terms:

1. testopathy _____
2. prostatodynia _____
3. oscheoplasty _____
4. epididymectomy _____
5. orchialgia _____
6. seminal _____
7. orchiepididymitis _____
8. gynecopathy _____
9. oogenesis _____
10. oophorotomy _____
11. intrauterine _____
12. metromalacia _____
13. vaginoplasty _____
14. colpodynia _____
15. hysteroscopy _____

Practice 5.22 Write a medical term for each of the following definitions:

1. excision of the testes _____
2. surgical repair of glans penis _____
3. incision of the renal pelvis _____
4. fixation of the bladder _____
5. difficult urination _____
6. narrowing of the urethra _____
7. suturing of the perineum _____
8. herniation of the uterus _____
9. puncture of the amnion _____
10. rupture of an ovary _____

Table 5.20 Abbreviations Used for the Male and Female Reproductive Systems

Abbreviation	Meaning
AB	abortion
AFP	alpha-fetoprotein
AH	abdominal hysterectomy
AI	aromatase inhibitor
BNO	bladder neck obstruction
BPH	benign prostatic hyperplasia
BRCA1	breast cancer gene 1
BSE	breast self-examination
BV	bacterial vaginosis
CIN	cervical intraepithelial neoplasia

Table 5.20 Abbreviations Used for the Male and Female Reproductive Systems—Cont'd

Abbreviation	Meaning
CIS	carcinoma in situ
CS	cesarean section
D&C	dilation and curettage
DRE	digital rectal examination
DUB	dysfunctional uterine bleeding
EMB	endometrial biopsy
ERT	estrogen replacement therapy
FHT	fetal heart tones
FSH	follicle-stimulating hormone
FTND	full-term normal delivery
G	gravid
GC	gonococcus
GU	genitourinary
GYN	gynecology
HCG	human chorionic gonadotropin
HPV	human papillomavirus
HRT	hormone replacement therapy
HSV	herpes simplex virus
IUD	intrauterine device
IVF	in vitro fertilization
LBW	low birthweight
LH	luteinizing hormone
LMP	last menstrual period
NB	new born
OB	obstetrics
OCP	oral contraceptive pill
PID	pelvic inflammatory disease
PMP	previous menstrual period
PMS	premenstrual syndrome
PSA	prostate genetic antigen
STD	sexually transmitted disease
STI	sexually transmitted infection
TAH-BSO	total abdominal hysterectomy with bilateral salpingo-oophorectomy
TRAM	transverse rectus abdominis muscle
TSE	testicular self-examination
TSS	toxic shock syndrome
TURP	transurethral resection of the prostate gland
TVH	total vagina hysterectomy
UC	uterine contractions
UTI	urinary tract infection
VD	venereal disease
VDRL	venereal disease research laboratory

11. The **immune system** is composed of a network of cells such as the white blood cells, tissues, and organs that function together in order to protect the body from organisms such as bacteria, parasites, and fungi that may cause infection and diseases. The immune system consists of the bone marrow, thymus, spleen, and lymph nodes. All blood cells are produced in the bone marrow through a process called hematopoiesis.

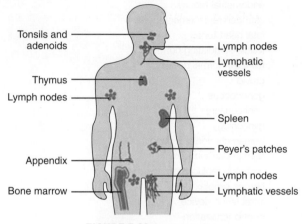

FIGURE 5.23 Immune system.

Table 5.21 Roots for the Immune System

Root	Meaning	Example	Meaning
blast/o	embryonic cell	erythroblastosis	abnormal increase of embryonic cells
immun/o	immunity	immunization	production of immunity
kary/o	nucleus	karyolysis	destruction of the nucleus
lymph/o	lymphocyte	lymphocytic	pertaining to lymphocytes
lymphaden/o	lymph gland	lymphadenopathy	disease of lymph nodes
myel/o	bone marrow	myelogenous	originating in the bone marrow
phag/o	swallowing	phagocyte	cell that is capable of engulfing bacteria and other things
ser/o	serum	serology	study of serum
splen/o	spleen	splenorrhagia	bursting forth of the spleen
thym/o	thymus gland	thymopathy	any disease of the thymus gland

Practice 5.23 Write the proper medical term for each of the following definitions:

1. tumor of the thymus _____
2. lacking in some immune function _____
3. cell of a gland _____
4. enlargement of the spleen _____
5. inflammation of the lymph glands _____

Table 5.22 Abbreviations Used for the Immune System	
Abbreviation	**Meaning**
AIDS	acquired immunodeficiency virus
HIV	human immunodeficiency virus
IgA	immunoglobulin A
IgD	immunoglobulin D
IgE	immunoglobulin E
IgG	immunoglobulin G
IgM	immunoglobulin M
SLE	systemic lupus erythematosus

FOCUS ON READING

Read the following passage and answer the questions that follow:

1. The ethical and legal principle of confidentiality is anchored in a set of values and assumptions about the treatment relationship and the consequences of disclosing private information. In the context of treating mental illness, these values include the following.
2. First, confidentiality is considered important because of the continuing **stigma** that is often associated with seeking mental health treatment. Until the late 1960s, the law often endorsed discrimination against people with mental illness. Because a diagnosis of mental illness was often equated with incompetence in decision making, treatment could result in the loss of key civil rights, including the right to enter into a contractual relationship, the right to vote, and the right to execute a will. Although these legal consequences have generally disappeared, mental illness still may cause negative consequences for the individual. For example, it is worth noting that before the recent political preoccupation with sexual issues, a way of **discrediting** an opponent politically was to reveal that he or she had been treated for mental illness. Examples included the attempted theft of Daniel Ellsberg's psychiatric records after he disclosed the

Pentagon Papers; the removal of Senator Thomas Eagleton from the Democratic ticket in 1972 after it was revealed that he had undergone electroshock treatment for depression; and the distribution of the treatment records of a Congressional candidate who had been treated for depression to the media during the 1992 elections.

3. Confidentiality is also considered important in creating trust in the clinical relationship. Many mental health professionals assume that mental health treatment is most likely to be successful only when the client trusts the clinician. The United States Supreme Court endorsed this assumption in a recent case creating a psychotherapeutic privilege in federal court proceedings. The Court wrote that:

"Effective psychotherapy depends upon an atmosphere of confidence and trust in which the patient is willing to make a frank and complete disclosure of facts, emotions, memories, and fears. Because of the sensitive nature of the problems for which individuals consult psychotherapists, disclosure of confidential communications made during counseling sessions may cause embarrassment or disgrace. For this reason, the mere possibility of disclosure may impede development of the confidential relationship necessary for successful treatment."

4. The creation of trust as a predicate for treatment may be particularly important when the prescribed treatment consists of verbal therapies in which the person is asked to be as unguarded as possible. Disclosures in this context, described by one commentator as "confessional" in nature, may be particularly important to protect because **they** often reveal material that is fundamentally private.

5. Confidentiality also advances the related values of privacy and autonomy. In the past three decades, the law has given increased weight to the value of privacy, while expanding individual autonomy in health care decision making. Confidentiality is important because of its assurance that individuals will have privacy in the health care relationship, which in turn may increase the likelihood that people will exercise autonomy by seeking needed treatment.

6. Research suggests that these assumptions have at least some empiric footing. For example, a number of studies suggest that the relative strength of confidentiality protections can play an important role in individual decisions to seek or forgo mental health and substance abuse treatment. In particular, the willingness of a person to make the self-disclosures necessary to such mental health and substance abuse treatment may decrease as the perceived negative consequences of a breach of confidentiality increase.

A. **Circle the correct answer.**

  1. Discrediting political candidates could be done by
     a. uncovering details about his/her mental illness
     b. treating the candidate's mental illness
     c. accusing him/her of stealing money
     d. paying candidate to leave the campaign

2. As stated in this text, disclosing information about clients could be considered
   a. professional
   b. confessional
   c. normal
   d. embarrassing
3. Autonomy is closest in meaning to
   a. privacy
   b. strength
   c. independence
   d. team decision

B. **True or false**
   1. _____ A diagnosis for mental illness could be a sufficient excuse to prevent someone from running elections.
   2. _____ The removal of Senator Thomas Eagleton from the Democratic ticket in 1972 was the result of disclosing confidential information.
   3. _____ Disclosing confidential information is necessary for successful treatment.
   4. _____ A person may reveal more information about his/her mental health if the level of confidentiality decreases.
   5. _____ Confidentiality may lead to the development of privacy, another desired value.

C. **Complete the following sentences.**
   1. The pronoun **they** in paragraph 4 refers to _____.
   2. The word **stigma** in paragraph 2 means _____.
   3. The word **discrediting** in paragraph 2 means _____.
   4. **Paragraph 5** is about the relationship between _____.
   5. The best title for this passage may be _____.

D. **Word building:** Complete the following table as required.

Adverb	Adjective	Noun	Verb
		confidence	
		communication	
x			endorse
x		disclosure	
		embarrassment	
			perceive
	effective		
mentally			x

VOCABULARY DEVELOPMENT

Collocations: Medical Idioms

1. **live and kicking:** alive and healthy
   How are feeling today, Jack? I am still live and kicking.
2. **a bitter pill to swallow:** an unpleasant fact that one must accept
   Losing the election was a bitter pill to swallow for the candidate.
3. **clean bill of health:** a report or certificate that a person or animal is healthy
   My doctor gave me a clean bill of health when I visited him last month.
4. **in labor:** a woman going through childbirth
   My friend's wife was in labor for 10 h.
5. **prescription-strength:** so strong that you need a doctor's written permission to buy it
   The patient needs a prescription-strength **ointment** to get rid of that rash.
6. **in remission:** a disease that seems to be getting better
   The cancer of my neighbor's mother has been in remission for several months.
7. **feel on top of the world:** to feel very healthy
   I have been feeling on top of the world since I quit smoking.
8. **checkup:** an examination of a patient by a doctor
   I plan to have my annual checkup next week.
9. **under the weather:** not feeling well
   My boss has been under the weather all week and has not come to work during that time.
10. **splitting headache:** a severe headache
    I have been suffering from a splitting headache for a couple of days.
11. **run down:** in poor physical condition
    The farmer is completely run down from lack of proper food.
12. **in the pink of health:** in excellent physical condition
    The employee looks in the pink of health after his holiday.
13. **out of sorts:** upset and irritable or not feeling well
    The baby is out of sorts today. Perhaps he is cutting a tooth.
14. **off color:** look or feel ill
    What is the matter with the teacher? He looks a bit off color today.
15. **in bad shape:** in poor physical condition
    I am really in bad shape. I must do more exercise.
16. **hang out one's shingle:** give public notice of the opening of a doctor's office, etc.
    The doctor decided to hang up his shingle as soon as he finished medical school.

17. **head shrinker:** a psychiatrist
    The man was advised to see a head shrinker after he threatened his wife several times.
18. **on the mend:** healing, becoming better
    My grandmother is on the mend after she broke her arm last week.
19. **vim and vigor:** have lots of vitality, energy, and enthusiasm
    After a relaxing holiday, the students came back to school full of vim and vigor.
20. **fill a prescription:** to get medicine from a pharmacy according to the orders of a doctor
    The patient went to a drugstore to fill a prescription.

Practice 5.24 Circle the idiom that replaces the words/phrases in bold in each of the following questions.

1. The doctor **announced the opening of his new clinic** immediately after passing the required examinations.
   a. hang out his shingle
   b. drawing blood
   c. at death's door
   d. going under the knife
2. After walking home in the rain, I **became sick** with a cold.
   a. on the mend
   b. off color
   c. took a turn for the worse
   d. blacked out
3. The worker is **in poor physical condition** due to malnutrition.
   a. back on his feet
   b. under the weather
   c. breathing his last
   d. run down
4. Our secretary is **becoming better** after she broke her arm.
   a. over the worst
   b. getting a splitting headache
   c. under the weather
   d. on the mend
5. Although the man was very sick, I think that he is now **in an excellent condition**.
   a. off sorts
   b. in the pink of health
   c. pulling through
   d. in remission

6. I went to the doctor last week and got a **medical checkup**.
   a. ran a temperature
   b. had a physical
   c. felt on top of the world
   d. went under the knife

7. After eating the seafood at the small restaurant, I suffered from a **severe pain in the head.**
   a. had a splitting headache
   b. felt out of sorts
   c. had a physical
   d. broke out

8. The patient was advised to see a **psychiatrist** after he began to act crazy at work.
   a. go to a head shrinker
   b. go under the knife
   c. breathe his last
   d. pull through

9. The doctor gave the boxer **a report that he was healthy** after he fainted and fell to the floor.
   a. a checkup
   b. a prescription-strength
   c. a run down
   d. a clean bill of health

10. The cancer of my friend's father has been **getting better** in the last 3 months.
    a. off sorts
    b. in bad shape
    c. in remission
    d. under the weather

Practice 5.25 Translate the following sentences into your own language paying attention to the use of idioms.

1. The doctor decided to **hang up his shingle** as soon as he finished medical school.
2. Our company sent all the employees **to have a physical** last week.
3. The man was advised to see **a head shrinker** after he threatened the woman in the store several times.
4. My grandfather is **on the mend** after he broke his leg last week.
5. My brother is **over the worst** since his skiing accident last month.
6. The car accident was very bad and I do not think that the driver will **pull through**.

7. The little boy is **running a temperature** and should stay in bed all day.
8. He was working very hard last month and has become very **run down**.
9. I have been suffering from **a splitting headache** all morning.
10. My aunt **took a turn for the worse** last week and is still in the hospital.
11. The nurse **took my temperature** when I went to the hospital yesterday.
12. The woman **threw up** several times after eating a bad fish.
13. My boss has been **feeling under the weather** all week and has not come to work during that time.

Academic Words

Study the following academic lists.

Academic List 1

Words	Definitions
1. stabilized	steady and not likely to move or change
2. challenge	something that tests strength, skill, or ability, especially in a way that is interesting
3. medicinal	relating to or having therapeutic properties
4. reject	to refuse, accept, believe in, or agree with something
5. expose	to put someone in a situation where they are not protected from something dangerous or unpleasant
6. network	a group of people, organizations, etc. that are connected or work together
7. academic	relating to institutionalized education and scholarship, especially at a college or university
8. compounds	a substance containing atoms from two or more elements
9. alter	to change, or to make someone or something change
10. decline (n)	a decrease in the quality, quantity, or importance of something

Academic List 2

Words	Definitions
1. instructive	providing a lot of useful information
2. expand	to become larger in size, number, or amount, or to make something become larger
3. allocate	to decide officially that a particular amount of money, time, etc. should be used for a particular purpose
4. enhance	to improve the quality or value of something
5. explicit	expressed in a way that is very clear and direct
6. recovery	the process of getting better after an illness, injury
7. enable	to make it possible for someone to do something, or for something to happen
8. discriminate	to recognize a difference between things

Words	Definitions
9. incidence	the number of times something happens, especially crime, disease, etc.
10. interval	the period of time between two events, activities

Practice 5.26 Match the words in column A with their definitions in column B by writing the letter of the correct answer next to the word in column A.

A	B
1. network _____	a. the number of times something happens, especially crime, disease, etc.
2. medicinal _____	b. a decrease in the quality, quantity, or importance of something
3. alter _____	c. to become larger in size, number, or amount, or to make something become larger
4. stabilized _____	d. the period of time between two events, activities
5. decline _____	e. relating to or having therapeutic properties
6. expand _____	f. to recognize a difference between things
7. instructive _____	g. steady and not likely to move or change
8. discriminate _____	h. providing a lot of useful information
9. incidence _____	i. to change, or to make someone or something change
10. intervals _____	j. a group of people, organizations, etc. that are connected or that work together

Practice 5.27 Complete each of the following sentences using the correct word from the box.

compounds	challenge	medicinal	reject	exposed
network	academic	stabilized	altered	decline

1. The old man was seriously ill when he was first admitted to hospital, but his condition has since _____.
2. There is a _____ of scientists working throughout the world to find a cure for cancer.
3. She got sick and missed most of the _____ year, so there was no way she could pass.
4. Modernization has been associated with a _____ in the status of the elderly.
5. Ana has cancer but she is ready to face this _____ and fight for her life.
6. Chemical analysis of chromosomes shows that they consist of four basic _____.

7. She uses a variety of _____ herbs to treat her illnesses.
8. The chemical balance of the brain which controls awareness can be radically _____ by the introduction of external agents.
9. Studies show that children who are _____ to tobacco smoke at home have more ear infections, and other health problems.
10. He received a heart transplant, and had to take drugs for the rest of his life so that his body would not _____ it.

Practice 5.28 Complete each of the following sentences using the correct word from the box.

instructive	expands	allocates	enhance	explicit
recovery	intervals	enable	discriminate	incidence

1. Young people need _____ information about sex, in order to avoid unwanted pregnancies or sexually transmitted infections.
2. During pregnancy, a woman's uterus _____ to 500 times its normal size.
3. New discoveries in genetics may someday _____ doctors to detect many inherited diseases before people actually develop them.
4. Billions of dollars have been spent on cancer research in the last 40 years, yet the _____ of cancer continues to increase.
5. Changing your attitude from negative to positive may _____ your physical health.
6. The findings of this study are quite _____ and should be very helpful in helping us decide the best treatment for the disease.
7. The patient had to be woken at regular _____ to take his medicine.
8. Doctors believe my mother's quick _____ from her illness was partly due to her desire to see her grandchildren again.
9. The new budget _____ an increase of over a billion dollars to the Ministry of Health.
10. This new drug is able to _____ between healthy cells and cancerous cells, and only attacks the cancerous cells.

FOCUS ON GRAMMAR

Phrasal verbs are very common in spoken and written English. A phrasal verb consists of a verb plus a particle (adverb) or a preposition. The meaning of a phrasal verb is different from the combined meanings of its components. It is necessary for health care professionals to have an adequate level of mastery of the most common phrasal verbs used in their careers.

The following is a list of some common phrasal verbs used in the various health care fields.

1. **cut down on**: *to reduce something*
   Consuming too much sugar may cause obesity and type 2 diabetes. If you want to be healthy, you have to *cut down on* sweets before it is too late.

2. **come down with (something)**: *to become sick, to catch an illness*
   My friend came down with the flu last week and cancelled his trip to China.

3. **phase out**: *to gradually stop using something*
   The use of this medicine will be phased out for the next 2 years.

4. **get rid of something**: *to eliminate it*
   The doctor advised the patient to use a better lotion to get rid of the rashes on his body.

5. **pull through**: *to recover from a serious illness, to survive*
   The car accident was very bad and I do not think that the driver will pull through.

6. **pass away**: *to die*
   The cancer patient passed away after a long period of treatment.

7. **bring up something/bring something up**: *vomit*
   The fish was not cooked properly and as soon as he ate it, he brought it up.

8. **pack up**: *to stop functioning*
   The doctor advised the patient to stop smoking; otherwise, his lungs will pack up in 2 years.

9. **get over something**: *become better after being ill, recover from being sick*
   The director will resume work as soon as he gets over the flu.

10. **pass out**: *faint, lose consciousness*
    The room was so hot and stuffy that he passed out.

11. **come round**: *recover consciousness after fainting or being unconscious*
    The old man fainted but came round again after we opened a window and got some fresh air into the room.

12. **build up your strength**: *become stronger, or to make someone or something do this*
    The patient has had the flu and has not eaten for days. She needs to build up her strength before she can go back to work.

13. **put on weight**: *increase in weight, to get fatter or heavier*
    I really need to go on a diet. I put so much weight on over the holidays.

14. **give birth**: *to have a baby*
    That lady gave birth to a baby girl last night.

15. **cut out something**: *stop eating or drinking something, usually to improve your health*
    He must **cut out sweets and chocolates** in order to lose weight.

16. **burn (oneself) out**: *to become very tired and almost sick from doing something for a long time or from working too hard*
After working long hours for many months, the woman finally burned herself out.

17. **have a physical (examination)**: *to get a medical checkup*
Our company sent all the employees to have a physical last week.

18. **lapse into a coma**: *to go into a coma*
The driver lapsed into a coma soon after the accident.

19. **nurse (someone) back to health**: *to give someone care to restore him or her to good health*
My friend spent 3 weeks with his grandmother trying to nurse her back to health.

20. **run in the family**: *to be a common family characteristic*
The serious illness runs in the family of my friend.

21. **refill a prescription**: *to sell/buy a second set of medicine on a doctor's orders*
I went to the pharmacy to refill a prescription for my mother.

22. **patch someone up**: *to give basic medical help to someone injured*
He was bleeding badly but nurses managed to patch him up temporarily.

23. **go down with something** : *to become ill*
My grandmother went down with the flu 2 weeks ago and her immune system is still recovering.

24. **break out with something** : *to start suddenly (e.g., a disease or a rash)*
The young girl broke out with a rash due to her nut allergy.

25. **look into something**: *to examine something*
I cannot say anything at this moment. I need to look into the patient's family disease history.

26. **black out**: *lose consciousness, faint*
The driver blacked out after the accident.

Practice 5.29 Circle the correct answer.

1. The patient is trying hard to **get rid of** his illness.
   - a. fight off
   - b. pick up
   - c. go down with
   - d. tide over
2. Another expression for **vomiting** is to
   - a. throw up
   - b. toss out
   - c. pass out
   - d. flare up
3. To become unconscious is to
   - a. go out
   - b. black out
   - c. knock over
   - d. burn out

4. The nurses were able to **patch up** all the injured people in the accident.
   a. give basic medical help
   b. move to hospital
   c. regain consciousness
   d. examine thoroughly
5. He must **cut out** rice and fries in order to lose weight.
   a. work out   b. reduce
   c. quit   d. toss out
6. To **become very tired and almost sick** from doing something for a long time or from working too hard is to
   a. work out oneself
   b. burn out oneself
   c. pull through
   d. black out
7. **To lose consciousness** is to
   a. break out
   b. sleep long
   c. go down with something
   d. lapse into coma
8. The use of this drug will be **phased out** in the next couple of years.
   a. continue to be used
   b. discontinued
   c. replaced
   d. modified
9. The surgeon advised the smoker to quit smoking; otherwise, his lungs will **pack up** in less than 3 years.
   a. continue functioning
   b. swell up
   c. stop functioning
   d. come round
10. The two brothers **broke out with** chickenpox at the same time.
   a. got it suddenly
   b. got it gradually
   c. recovered from it
   d. transmitted it

ORAL COMMUNICATION SKILLS

Read the following dialogue with a classmate.

Patient: Good afternoon.
Doctor: Good afternoon. Have a seat. What have you come in for today?

Patient: Thank you. I don't feel well. I've got a bad cough, and I have a fever as well.

Doctor: I see. How long have you had these symptoms?

Patient: Oh, I've had the cough for 3 weeks. It has come worse in the last 3 days.

Doctor: Are you having any other problems?

Patient: Well, I've got a headache. I've also had a little bit of diarrhea.

Doctor: Do you produce any phlegm when coughing?

Patient: Sometimes, but it's usually pretty dry.

Doctor: Do you smoke?

Patient: Yes, a few cigarettes a day. No more than 10 cigarettes a day.

Doctor: How about allergies? Do you have any allergies to food?

Patient: Not that I'm aware of.

Doctor: Does your head feel stuffy?

Patient: Yes, for the past few days.

Doctor: OK. Now let's have a look. Could you please open your mouth and say "ah"?

Doctor: It seems that you have throat infection. Your tonsils are a little bit swollen. I will give an injection and some medicines. You also need to gargle with salt and warm water three times a day. I hope that you will feel better within 3 days.

Patient: Thank you doctor. I will follow your advice.

Doctor: If you don't get better within 4 days, you need to see me again.

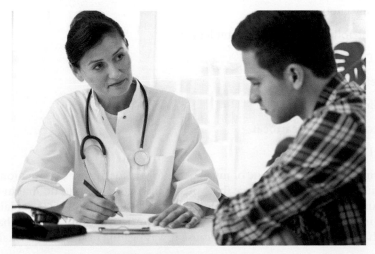

FIGURE 5.24 A doctor and his patient.

Practice 5.30 Act out the dialogue.

Use the following terms or phrases in sentences of your own.
1. to feel ill
2. to have a cough
3. phlegm
4. allergy
5. to feel stuffy
6. headache

FOCUS ON WRITING

Referral letters

Very often doctors need to refer their patients to certain specialists for more advanced checkups and investigation. When you need to write a referral letter, you need to follow the following steps:
1. Greet the specialist and indicate which specialization you are referring your patient to.
2. Introduce your patient and his/her case. State the patient's personal information including his/her name, age, date of birth, gender, and contact details. State why are you referring him/her to this doctor. Include the patient's medical details.
3. Explain how you came to know the patient, for how long, and in what circumstances.
4. Conclude the letter by informing the specialist that you are available for any enquiry.

Read the following sample referral letter.

Dear Dr Mathews,

217 Jefferson Street

Building 23, Apartment 12

Subject: **Irregular heartbeat**

Dear Dr Mathews,

Greetings! I am referring one of my patients to you for further examination and treatment of his heart. I believe that you are the right person to do that in light of your good reputation as a cardiologist. Mr Jack visited my clinic complaining of a tingling sensation in his hands and chest. After checkup, I found that he may have a problem in his heart because it was beating faster than normal.

Mr Jack is a 45-year-old male who was born on March 2, 1972. He may be contacted through his home phone number . . . or through his mobile phone number . . ., although he prefers to be contacted through his mobile phone number.

I will be glad to answer any questions that you may have regarding his case. You can contact me through my work phone number . . . .

Best regards,

Dr James Lyon

3rd Ave. Bldg. 24, Apartment 10

Practice 5.31 Imagine that you are a GP and you need to refer one of your patients to an oncologist. Write a letter to refer this patient to an oncologist.

PRONUNCIATION OF MEDICAL TERMS

The following are the medical terms introduced in this chapter. You are supposed to read them aloud as many times as you need to master their pronunciation. In this activity, you are also required to give the meaning of each term in order to retain them active in your memory.

Read the following medical terms and know their meanings.

acetabulectomy	arteriosclerosis
acromial	arthritis
adenoid	asynovia
adenoidectomy	atherosclerosis
adenopathy	audiometer
adiposis	aural
adrenocorticotropic	auriculocranial
adrenomegaly	balanitis
alveolitis	biliary
amblyopia	blepharoptosis
amniocentesis	brachialgia
anal	bradykinesia
angiogram	bronchiolectasis
ankylosis	bronchitis
anthracosis	buccogingival
aortic stenosis	calcaneodynia
aphakia	calioplasty
appendectomy	calicectomy
appendicitis	capnogram
arteriolitis	cardiology

cardiovascular
carpoptosis
cecoptosis
celioma
cephalad
cerebral
ceruminolytic
cervical
cervicitis
cheiloplasty
cholangioma
cholecystectomy
choledochotomy
cholestasis
clavicular
clitorectomy
coccygeal
cochleitis
colostomy
colonoscopy
colpostenosis
condylectomy
conjunctivoplasty
coreoplasty
corneoblepharon
coronary
corticospinal
craniotomy
cyclodialysis
cystitis
dacryorrhea
dactylitis
dermal
dermatology
duodenostomy
dysentery
dyslexia
dystocia
dystonia
edentulous
embolectomy
embryonic

encephalitis
epididymotomy
epiglottitis
episiotomy
ergograph
erythroblastosis
esophageal
extrapulmonary
fasciodesis
femoral
fetometry
fibulocalcaneal
galactopoiesis
ganglionectomy
gastrojejunostomy
gastroscopy
gingivitis
glioma
glomerulitis
glossoplegia
glucogenesis
glycolysis
gonadotropin
gynecologist
hemangioma
hepatitis
hidradenitis
humeroscapular
hypophyseal
hysterectomy
ichthyosis
ileitis
iliac
immunization
inosclerosis
insular
interatrial
intervertebral
intravenous
intraventricular
iridocele
iridopupillary

ischiodynia
karyolysis
keratolysis
kinesis
kinesitherapy
kyphosis
labium
labyrinthitis
lacrimotomy
lactogenesis
laminectomy
laryngoscope
leiomyoma
lentiform
leptomeningopathy
ligamentous
lingual
lipocele
lithotripsy
lobectomy
lordosis
lumbar
lymphadenopathy
lymphangitis
lymphocyte
lymphocytic
lymphoma
mammography
mastitis
mastoiditis
maxillofacial
meatotomy
mediastinitis
medullary
melanocyte
meningococci
menopause
metacarpectomy
metropathy
endometrium
muscular
mycology

myelgenous
myelitis
myocardial
myositis
myringotomy
narcosis
nasal
nephrologist
neuroplasty
ocular
onychomalacia
oocyte
oophorectomy
oophoritis
ophthalmologist
optometer
oral
orchiopexy
orchidectomy
orchitis
oropharynx
orthodontics
orthopedist
oscheal
ossiculectomy
osteoma
otitis
ovarian cyst
ovariopexy
ovoid
ovulatory
oximeter
palatine
palpebral
pancreatitis
parathyroidectomy
patellectomy
pectoralgia
pedograph
peribursal
perinecele
perisacral

peritonitis
phagocyte
phalangeal
pharyngospasm
phlebitis
phonometer
phrenicotripsy
phrenitis
pilonidal
pleurocentesis
pneumoconiosis
pneumonia
pneumectomy
podiatry
polyspermia
prenatal
proctopexy
prognathic
prostatometer
psychoactive
pubococcygeal
pyelogram
pyloroplasty
rachiocentesis
radiculitis
rectocele
renal
retinitis
rhabdoid
rhabdomyoma
rhinoplasty
salpingitis
salpingoscope
sclerectasia
scoliosis
scotometer
seborrhea
septoplasty
septostomy
serology
sialoadenitis
sialogram

sigmoidoscopy
sinusotomy
somnolence
sphygmomanometer
spirometer
splenomegaly
splenorrhagia
spondylosis
steatorrhea
steatosis
sternad
stethoscope
subchondriac
subchoroidal
subcostal
subcutaneous
sudoresis
supracerebellar
suprapelvic
pelvioscope
supraventricular
tendinitis
tenodesis
testosterone
thalamotomy
thoracoschisis
thoracotomy
thrombocytosis
thymectomy
thymopathy
thyroadenitis
thyrotoxic
tibiafemoral
tonsillar
tonsillectomy
tracheotome
trichophagia
trigonitis
tympanoplasty
ulnocarpal
ungual
uremia

nocturia
ureterectasis
urethrostenosis
uteroplastsy
uveitis
uvulotome
vaginitis
valvar
valvuloplasty
varicocele

vasodepressor
vasostomy
venulitis
vesical
vesiculogram
vestibulotomy
vulvitis
xenograft
xeroderma
xerostomia

REVIEW EXERCISES

A. **Case study: Read the following case study and answer the questions following it.**

N.J., a 79-year-old man, was admitted to Al Qasimia Hospital on October 23, 2005. Prior to being admitted to the hospital, N.J. had been in excellent health. His troubles apparently began 3 weeks prior to being admitted. On October 23, N.J.'s son found him lying on the floor confused, and soaked in urine.

Mr J. was diagnosed as having an acute cerebral vascular accident. This disorder can also be described as a "stroke." It occurs when there is an interruption of normal blood flow in one or more of the blood vessels that supply the brain. Thrombosis, embolism, and hemorrhage are the primary causes of a CVA. The tissues of the brain become ischemic, leading to hypoxia or anoxia with destruction or necrosis of the neurons, glia, and vasculature. Complications of CVA include unstable blood pressure, sensory and motor impairment, infection, pneumonia, contractures, and pulmonary emboli. CVA is the third leading cause of death in the USA and affects more than 500,000 Americans annually.

He was widowed in November 2002. One of his daughters has coronary artery disease; one son died of an MI at age 35; the other one died with lung cancer at 52. N.J. had been the primary caregiver of his daughter until she was admitted to the hospital 3 weeks ago. She is dying with a short bowel syndrome and cirrhosis and is now being taken care of in hospice. Soon after being left alone, Mr N.J.'s appetite decreased and he had become congested. He was placed on Xanax to treat symptoms of depression. He had also been taking Augmentin for congestion. Also his family noticed that he was suffering from confusion. As a result, they brought him into the Emergency Room for evaluation. The Emergency Room doctors performed a CT scan of the brain which revealed evidence of old strokes. The doctors stopped the Augmentin and placed him on Z-pack. This seemed to improve his state of confusion, as well as reduce his symptoms of congestion.

On October 22, 2005, he was seen for the congestion. The doctor examined him thoroughly. This exam included giving him a chest X-ray. The chest X-ray proved to be normal. His white blood count was elevated and he was found to be mildly dehydrated. He was prescribed Amoxicillin 500 three times a day, and Guaifenesin. His past medical history is short including depression, stroke, and presbyacusis. He has not had any prior surgery and there are no known allergies.

I. Circle the best answer
1. Ischemic stroke is generally caused by
   a. hemorrhage
   b. hematoma
   c. thrombosis
   d. hemiparesis
2. Signs and symptoms that occur together are termed
   a. prodrome
   b. syndrome
   c. exacerbation
   d. remission

II. Write a medical term from the case study for each of the following meanings:
1. obstruction or occlusion of a blood vessel _____
2. coagulation of the blood within a blood vessel in any part of the circulatory system _____
3. pertaining to the lungs _____
4. the condition of being unable to perform as a consequence of physical or mental unfitness _____
5. deficiency in the amount of oxygen reaching body tissues _____
6. the delicate web of connective tissue that surrounds and supports nerve cells _____
7. an acute or chronic disease marked by inflammation of the lungs _____
8. a liver disease in which normal liver cells are gradually replaced by scar tissue, causing the organ to shrink, harden, and lose its function _____

III. What does each of the following abbreviations stand for:
   a. CVA _____
   b. CT _____
   c. CAD _____

IV. Describe orally the case of N.J. briefly.
V. Name three medicines he was given.

B. **Answer the following questions.**

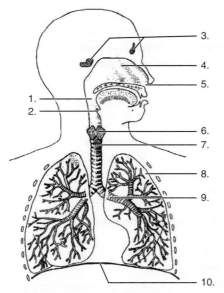

1. Identify the organ/structure at number 1.
   a. larynx
   b. pharynx
   c. epiglottis
   d. sinuses

2. Identify the structure at number 2.
   a. pharynx
   b. larynx
   c. trachea
   d. epiglottis

3. Identify the structure at number 3.
   a. pharynx
   b. sinuses
   c. epiglottis
   d. external nares

4. Identify the structure at number 4.
   a. external nares
   b. nasal passages
   c. sinuses
   d. pharynx

5. Identify the structure at number 5.
   a. external nares
   b. pharynx
   c. larynx
   d. sinuses

6. Identify the structure at number 6.
   a. larynx
   b. pharynx
   c. trachea
   d. bronchus
7. Identify the structure at number 7.
   a. larynx
   b. bronchus
   c. trachea
   d. epiglottis
8. Identify the structure at number 8.
   a. lung
   b. diaphragm
   c. epiglottis
   d. pharynx
9. Identify the structure at number 9.
   a. trachea
   b. bronchus
   c. epiglottis
   d. sinuses
10. Identify the organ/structure at number 10.
    a. larynx
    b. pharynx
    c. epiglottis
    d. diaphragm

C. Circle the correct answer.

1. All of the following are basic tissue types, except
   a. muscle tissue
   b. epithelial tissue
   c. nervous tissue
   d. bone tissue
2. Morphology is the study of
   a. metabolism
   b. energy
   c. form
   d. chemicals
3. Cytogenesis is
   a. formation of cells
   b. division of the nucleus
   c. formation of proteins
   d. formation of fibers

4. A megakaryocyte is a cell with a large
   a. membrane
   b. nucleus
   c. cytoplasm
   d. wall

5. In adiposuria, the urine contains
   a. sugar
   b. carbohydrate
   c. protein
   d. fat

6. Another name for growth hormone is
   a. neoplasm
   b. acidophilin
   c. somatotropin
   d. gonadotropin

7. Steatorrhea is the discharge of
   a. digestive enzymes
   b. fats
   c. alcohol
   d. mucus

8. Lithotripsy is
   a. measurement of a calculi
   b. surgical removal of a stone
   c. crushing of a stone
   d. removal of a calculi

9. Arthroplasty is
   a. measurement of a joint
   b. fusion of a joint
   c. surgery on the ear
   d. plastic repair of a joint

10. In gastropexy, the stomach is
    a. widened
    b. surgically fixed
    c. dilated
    d. stapled for weight loss

11. In a hepatorrhapy, the liver is
    a. divided
    b. drained
    c. stained
    d. repaired

12. A sphygmomanometer is used to measure
    a. pulse
    b. temperature
    c. sounds
    d. blood pressure
13. A small vein is a/an
    a. lymphatic duct
    b. lymphatic capillary
    c. arteriole
    d. venule
14. Which of the following is not considered to be part of the lymphatic system?
    a. spleen
    b. tonsils
    c. nodes
    d. liver
15. Cardioptosis is
    a. downward displacement of the heart
    b. irregularity of a heartbeat
    c. rupture of the heart
    d. caridomyopathy
16. A valvotome is a/an
    a. flap of a valve
    b. instrument for incising a valve
    c. instrument for measuring a valve
    d. cusp of a valve
17. Angiography is a/an
    a. X-ray study of vessels
    b. study of pressure in vessels
    c. X-ray study of the ventricles
    d. spasm of vessels
18. A term that means around a vessel is
    a. retrovascular
    b. isovascular
    c. supravascular
    d. perivascualr
19. A term that means within a vein is
    a. intervenous
    b. intravenous
    c. intervascular
    d. extravascular

20. Phlebectasia is
    a. constriction of a vein
    b. spasm of a vein
    c. dilation of a capillary
    d. dilation of a vein
21. Polyarteritis is
    a. constriction of two arteries
    b. inflammation of many arteries
    c. formation of tissue around arteries
    d. removal of tissue from an artery
22. Aortostenosis is
    a. dilation of the aorta
    b. narrowing of the aorta
    c. fissure of the aorta
    d. rupture of the aorta
23. Arteriosclerosis is
    a. widening of an artery
    b. growth of an artery
    c. shrinking of an arteriole
    d. hardening of an artery
24. Lymphadenopathy is
    a. inflammation of a lymphatic vessel
    b. removal of a lymph node
    c. any disease of a lymph node
    d. shrinking of a lymph node
25. Asplenia is
    a. enlargement of the spleen
    b. hardening of the spleen
    c. absence of the spleen
    d. resection of the spleen
26. A lymphocyte is a
    a. lymph node
    b. cell found in the lymphatic system
    c. cell that migrates to the heart
    d. location within the lymphatic system
27. A lymphangioma is a/an
    a. tumor of lymph nodes
    b. inflammation of lymphatic vessels
    c. tumor of lymphatic vessels
    d. removal of lymph nodes
28. The root in ischemia means
    a. heart
    b. lack
    c. hardening
    d. blood

29. Thrombosis is
    a. transportation of lipids in the blood
    b. formation of a blood clot
    c. an increase in blood supply
    d. a tumor of a lymph node
30. Phonocardiography is a/an
    a. photograph of the heart in action
    b. recording of heart sounds
    c. X-ray study of the heart
    d. study of the heart using a catheter
31. The abbreviation CPR stands for
    a. cardiovascular resuscitation
    b. chronic pulmonary resuscitation
    c. cardiopulmonary resuscitation
    d. creatine phosphoreaction
32. The abbreviation ECG stands for
    a. electrocardiogram
    b. elevated creatine glutamine
    c. electrocardiovascular
    d. elevated coronary enzymes
33. Erythropoiesis is
    a. formation of white cells
    b. formation of red cells
    c. destruction of red cells
    d. formation of platelets
34. A leukoblast is a/an
    a. immature platelet
    b. immature thrombocyte
    c. mature white blood cell
    d. immature white blood cell
35. The term *myelogenous* means
    a. deficiency of blood
    b. deficiency of bone marrow
    c. excess platelets in the blood
    d. originating in bone marrow
36. The membrane that covers the lungs is
    a. tonsil
    b. phrenic
    c. pleura
    d. glottis
37. The pharyngeal tonsils are also called the
    a. bronchi
    b. wheeze
    c. rhonchi
    d. adenoids

38. The epiglottis is the
    a. lower end of the trachea
    b. throat
    c. cartilage around the bronchioles
    d. cartilage that covers the trachea during swallowing
39. The scientific name for the throat is
    a. trachea
    b. larynx
    c. epiglottis
    d. pharynx
40. The muscle under the lungs is the
    a. palate
    b. cannula
    c. diaphragm
    d. sphincter
41. The nerve that activates the diaphragm is
    a. diaphragmatic
    b. carotid
    c. mediastinal
    d. phrenic
42. Bronchiectasis is
    a. constriction of the bronchi
    b. inflammation of the bronchi
    c. dilation of the bronchioles
    d. dilation of the bronchi
43. An endotracheal polyp is located
    a. below the trachea
    b. outside the trachea
    c. near the trachea
    d. within the trachea
44. Pleurocentesis is
    a. surgical puncture of the lungs
    b. excision of the pleura
    c. pain in the lungs
    d. surgical puncture of the pleura
45. Pneumonopathy is
    a. study of respiration
    b. study of the lungs
    c. faulty development of the lungs
    d. any disease of the lungs
46. A spirogram is a/an
    a. X-ray examination of the lungs
    b. record of lung measurements
    c. measurement of the pleura
    d. record of breathing measurements

47. Stomatosis is any disease of the
    a. stomach
    b. pylorus
    c. hepatic flexure
    d. mouth
48. The term *glossolabial* refers to
    a. tongue and lips
    b. palate and gums
    c. uvula and salivary gland
    d. lips and cheek
49. A term that means within the cheek
    a. supragingival
    b. intrabuccal
    c. buccogingival
    d. gnatholabial
50. Radiographic study of the salivary glands and ducts is
    a. glossography
    b. palatoplasty
    c. labiometry
    d. sialography
51. The term *perioral* means
    a. above the nose
    b. within the sinuses
    c. around the mouth
    d. around the jaw
52. An enterovirus infects the
    a. mouth
    b. throat
    c. tonsils
    d. intestine
53. Duodenoscopy is
    a. endoscopic examination of the appendix
    b. endoscopic examination of the first part of the small intestine
    c. resection of the small portion of the small intestine
    d. formation of an opening into the pancreas
54. Surgical creation of an opening into the middle portion of the small intestine is a/an
    a. jejunostomy
    b. ileostomy
    c. cecoduodenostomy
    d. jejunectomy

55. Inflammation of the ileum is
    a. ileumitis
    b. ileitis
    c. iliitis
    d. ileosis
56. Proctopexy is
    a. surgical repair of the sigmoid colon
    b. irrigation of the rectum
    c. surgical fixation of the rectum
    d. plastic repair of the anus
57. Cholangiography is
    a. a radiographic study of the gallbladder
    b. an X-ray image of the liver
    c. a radiographic study of the bile ducts
    d. the presence of bile in the blood
58. In pancreatolysis
    a. a biopsy specimen is taken from the pancreas
    b. bile is regurgitated
    c. the pancreas is excised
    d. pancreatic tissue is destroyed
59. Something that is harmful to the kidney is described as
    a. nephrotome
    b. postrenal
    c. nephritic
    d. nephrotoxic
60. Pyelectasis is
    a. lysis of the renal pelvis
    b. swelling of the calyx
    c. dilation of the upper part of the ureter
    d. softening of the renal medulla
61. Ureteropyeloplasty is
    a. excision of the renal pelvis
    b. surgical fixation of the ureter
    c. plastic repair of the ureter and renal pelvis
    d. inflammation of the renal pelvis
62. The root in the term *prevesical* means
    a. urination
    b. glomerulus
    c. iliac artery
    d. urinary bladder
63. A cystocele is a
    a. dilation of the bladder
    b. shrinking of the bladder
    c. dropping of the bladder
    d. hernia of the bladder

64. The sex glands are the
    a. spermatozoa
    b. androgens
    c. gonads
    d. glans

65. The epididymis is a
    a. type of cell that secrets semen
    b. hormone active in reproduction
    c. coiled tube on the testis that stores sperm cells
    d. cord that aids in the descent of the testis

66. Orchialgia is
    a. Pain in the prostate
    b. narrowing of the epididymis
    c. pain in the testis
    d. pain in the seminal vesicle

67. Excess secretion of semen is
    a. polyspermia
    b. multisemia
    c. oligospermia
    d. spermatopenia

68. Destruction of sperm cells is
    a. spermaturia
    b. spermatogenesis
    c. semispermia
    d. spermatolysis

69. An oscheolith is a/an
    a. sclerosis of the scrotum
    b. inflammation of the epididymis
    c. stone in the scrotum
    d. overgrowth of the prostate

70. Vesiculotomy is
    a. removal of the seminal vesicle
    b. incision of the ejaculatory duct
    c. suture of the scrotum
    d. incision of the seminal vesicle

71. Surgical fixation of the testis is
    a. orchiopexy
    b. orchiostomy
    c. spermatopexy
    d. spermatosis

72. Benign prostatic hyperplasia is
    a. removal of the prostate
    b. measurement of the prostate
    c. ultrasound study of the prostate
    d. enlargement of the prostate

73. The endometrium is the
    a. muscular layer of the uterus
    b. membrane that covers the outside of the uterus
    c. lining of the uterus
    d. upper portion of the vagina
74. A laparoscope is induced into the body
    a. through a vein
    b. through the vagina
    c. rectally
    d. through the abdominal wall
75. Oogenesis is
    a. formation of an egg cell
    b. fertilization of an egg cell
    c. rupture of an egg cell
    d. release of an egg cell from an ovary
76. Ovariorrhexis is
    a. dropping of an ovary
    b. repair of an ovary
    c. rupture of an ovary
    d. pain in an ovary
77. Any disease specific to women is
    a. gynecology
    b. gynecopathy
    c. gynodynia
    d. genealogy
78. Hysterotomy is
    a. removal of the cervix
    b. removal of the uterus
    c. surgical fixation of the uterus
    d. incision of the uterus
79. Vaginometry is
    a. hernia of the vagina
    b. rupture of the vagina
    c. measurement of the vagina
    d. radiography of the vagina
80. The term *uterovesical* refers to the
    a. vagina and cervix
    b. vagina and uterus
    c. uterus and urinary bladder
    d. urinary bladder and ovary
81. Colpectasia is
    a. dilation of the vagina
    b. dilation of the cervix
    c. constriction of the vagina
    d. surgical fixation of the uterus

82. Episiorrhaphy is
    a. plastic repair of the cul-de-sac
    b. removal of the cervix
    c. prolapse of the uterus
    d. suture of the vulva
83. Mastitis is
    a. inflammation of the clitoris
    b. absence of a breast
    c. absence of lactation
    d. inflammation of the breast
84. The endocrine glands secrete
    a. mucus
    b. serous fluid
    c. hormones
    d. saliva
85. Hypophysectomy is
    a. rupture of the hypophysis
    b. surgical removal of the pituitary gland
    c. ptosis of the pituitary gland
    d. endoscopic examination of the hypophysis
86. A parathyrotropic substance
    a. acts on the adrenal glands
    b. acts on the thyroid gland
    c. is attracted to the thymus gland
    d. acts on the parathyroid glands
87. A thyrolytic substance
    a. stimulates the thyroid gland
    b. destroys thyroid tissue
    c. interacts with the adrenal gland
    d. stimulates the thymus gland
88. Hernia of the meninges is
    a. a meningocele
    b. meningitis
    c. meningodysplasia
    d. a meningioma
89. A glioma is a/an
    a. tumor of the meninges
    b. inflammation of the spinal cord
    c. tumor of a ganglion
    d. tumor of neuroglia
90. A ganglionectomy is
    a. excision of a spinal nerve root
    b. surgical removal of a ganglion
    c. incision into a neuroglia
    d. pain in a nerve

91. Surgical creation of an opening into a brain ventricle is a
    a. ventricectomy
    b. ventriculitis
    c. ventriculoma
    d. ventriculostomy
92. The term *intacerebellar* means
    a. within the cerebrum
    b. between the brain stem and the cerebrum
    c. within the cerebellum
    d. between the cerebrum and the midbrain
93. Audiometry is measurement of
    a. taste
    b. hearing
    c. muscle strength
    d. vision
94. A myringotomy is the same as
    a. presbycusis
    b. tympanotomy
    c. stapedioplasty
    d. ophthalmology
95. The adjective lacrimal refers to
    a. taste
    b. odors
    c. sounds
    d. tears
96. Conjunctivitis affects the
    a. membrane that lines the eyelid
    b. layer of the eye between the retina and sclera
    c. layer of the eye between the retina and the choroid
    d. substance that fills the eyeball
97. Blepharospasm is
    a. drooping of the eyelid
    b. a stone in the tear duct
    c. paralysis of the eyelid
    d. sudden contraction of the eyelid
98. Keratoplasty is
    a. plastic repair of the uvea
    b. incision of the lens
    c. removal of the lacrimal apparatus
    d. plastic repair of the cornea
99. Retinoschisis is
    a. degeneration of the retina
    b. infection of the ciliary body
    c. prolapse of the retina
    d. splitting of the retina

100. An iridodilator
    a. narrows the pupil
    b. shortens the ciliary body
    c. widens the iris
    d. changes the color of the iris
101. The cranial bones are part of the
    a. sacrum
    b. sternum
    c. ribs
    d. skull
102. The cervical vertebrae are in the
    a. chest
    b. lower back
    c. upper back
    d. neck
103. Chondrogenesis is the formation of
    a. bone
    b. bone marrow
    c. cartilage
    d. synovial fluid
104. A bursolith is a/an
    a. stone in a bursa
    b. incision into a bursa
    c. region near a bursa
    d. repair of bursa
105. The term infracostal means
    a. within cartilage
    b. under a vertebra
    c. below the ribs
    d. above the coccyx
106. The sacroiliac joint is between the
    a. skull and first cervical vertebra
    b. zygomatic and temporal bones
    c. ribs and sternum
    d. spine and the pelvis
107. A coccygectomy is
    a. fracture of the coccyx
    b. malformation of the coccyx
    c. removal of the coccyx
    d. degeneration of the coccyx
108. In spondylolysis
    a. a rib is separated
    b. the pelvis ossifies
    c. the ilium is measured
    d. a vertebra is destroyed

109. The term *costochondral* refers to
    a. skull and spine
    b. rib and cartilage
    c. rib and vertebra
    d. cartilage and bone marrow

110. The acetabulum is
    a. the upper portion of the skull
    b. part of the intervertebral disk
    c. a socket in the hip bone
    d. the anterior joint of the pelvis

111. Tenotomy is
    a. tearing of a tendon
    b. movement of a tendon
    c. incision of a tendon
    d. splitting of a tendon

112. Dyskinesia is
    a. contraction of a muscle
    b. malformation of muscle fibers
    c. rapid movements
    d. abnormality of movement

113. The layer of the skin above the dermis is the
    a. subcutaneous layer
    b. sebaceous layer
    c. epidermis
    d. hypodermis

114. The subcutaneous layer is located
    a. above the dermis
    b. just below the epidermis
    c. along the shaft of a hair
    d. below the dermis

115. Hidradenitis is
    a. inflammation of a sweat gland
    b. infection of the hair
    c. inflammation of melanosomes
    d. loss of pigment

116. The term onychoid refers to a
    a. sebaceous gland
    b. follicle
    c. hair
    d. nail

117. Trichomycosis is a
    a. bacterial infection of a sweat gland
    b. bacterial infection of a nail
    c. fungal infection of hair
    d. viral infection of the epidermis

118. Keratogenesis is
    a. a tumor containing keratin
    b. formation of keratin
    c. destruction of keratin
    d. lysis of keratin
119. A word that means the same as subcutaneous is
    a. sudoriferous
    b. hypodermis
    c. hidrosis
    d. seborrheic
120. In hypohidrosis, one would expect
    a. reduced amount of sweat
    b. excess production of saliva
    c. reduced production of salivary enzymes
    d. excess release of sebum

D. What do the following medical abbreviations stand for?

1. OS _____
2. NVA _____
3. PERRLA _____
4. ROM _____
5. IM _____
6. TKA _____
7. ACS _____
8. ASHD _____
9. CABG _____
10. CPR _____
11. HDL _____
12. LV _____
13. HAART _____
14. SLE _____
15. CNS _____
16. ADHD _____
17. CSF _____
18. ALS _____
19. MRI _____
20. FSH _____
21. GTT _____
22. PGH _____
23. TSH _____
24. COLD _____
25. CPAP _____
26. IPPM _____
27. SIDS _____

28. RUL _____
29. BMI _____
30. ALT _____
31. CKD _____
32. CAPD _____
33. DRE _____
34. IVF _____
35. STD _____
36. TURP _____
37. VDRL _____
38. HIV _____
39. HD _____
40. ADH _____

E. **In each of the following sets, circle the word that does not fit with the rest and explain the reason for your choice.**

1	thoracic cavity	pelvic cavity	abdominal cavity	spinal cavity
2	lumb/o	dactyl/o	pod/o	brachi/o
3	thymus	tonsil	spleen	cusp
4	pancreas	gallbladder	liver	bronchial tube
5	ovary	pituitary	larynx	parathyroid
6	cutane/o	derm/o	kerat/o	myc/o
7	ossiculitis	hidradenitis	labyrinthitis	otitis
8	fibulocalcaneal	humeroscapular	valvuloplasty	spondylosis
9	phlebitis	angiogram	cardiovascular	vasodepressor
10	MI	NSR	CHF	CLL
11	meningococci	corticospinal	gonadotropin	supracerebellar
12	oophorectomy	pancreatomy	adenectomy	parathyroidectomy
13	alveolus	diaphragm	pleura	cecum
14	duodenum	jejunum	ilium	ileum
15	gloss/o	sigmoid/o	odont/o	gingiv/o
16	balanitis	orchiopexy	prostatometer	ovulatory

F. **Write T if the statement is true or F if it is false. Correct the false ones in the second blank.**
1. Myelogenous means originating in the spinal cord. _____ _____
2. Thrombocytopenia means deficiency of platelet in the blood. _____

   _____
3. A hematoma is a localized collection of blood. _____ _____
4. The vocal cords are located in the pharynx. _____ _____
5. Pyothorax is the accumulation of fluid in the chest. _____ _____

6. Above the diaphragm is termed superphrenic. _____ _____
7. From its name you might guess that the buccinators muscle is in the tongue. _____ _____
8. Hernia of the rectum is termed proctocele. _____ _____
9. Pyelitis is inflammation of the kidney. _____ _____
10. A lithotomy is an incision to remove a calculus. _____ _____
11. The adjective oscheal refers to the seminal vesicle. _____ _____
12. The lining of the uterus is the myometrium. _____ _____
13. Thyrolytic means destroying the thyroid glands. _____ _____
14. A narcotic is a drug that causes sleep. _____ _____
15. The cervical nerves are in the region of the neck. _____ _____
16. A myringotomy is incision of the vitreous body. _____ _____
17. Synovectomy is excision of bursa. _____ _____
18. The study of the efficient use of energy during work is termed ergonomics. _____ _____
19. To measure your blood pressure, you may use sphygmomanometer. _____ _____
20. Capnogram means record of breathing. _____ _____

G. **Define each of the following words, and give the meaning of the word parts in each.**
1. phonocardiography
    a. phon/o _____
    b. cardi/o _____
    c. -graphy _____
2. lymphangiophlebitis
    a. lymph/o _____
    b. angi/o _____
    c. phleb/o _____
    d. -itis _____
3. hemocytometer
    a. hem/o _____
    b. cyt/o _____
    c. -meter _____
4. intrapulmonary
    a. intra- _____
    b. pulmon/o _____
    c. -ary _____
5. supravesical
    a. supra- _____
    b. vesic/o _____
    c. -al _____

6. vesiculogram
   a. vesicul/o _____
   b. -gram _____
7. hysteropexy
   a. hyster/o _____
   b. -pexy _____
8. adenocorticotropic
   a. adenocortic/o _____
   b. -tropic _____
9. myelodysplasia
   a. myel/o _____
   b. dys- _____
   c. -plas _____
   d. -ia _____
10. polyneuroradiculitis
    a. poly- _____
    b. neur/o _____
    c. radicul/o _____
    d. -itis _____
11. circumcorneal
    a. circum- _____
    b. corne/o _____
    c. -eal _____
12. rachioschisis
    a. rachi/o _____
    b. -schisis _____
13. spondylosyndesis
    a. spondyl/o _____
    b. syn- _____
    c. -desis _____
14. amyotrophic
    a. a- _____
    b. my/o _____
    c. troph/o _____
    d. -ic _____
15. choledochotomy
    a. choledoch/o _____
    b. -tomy _____

H. Label each numbered part. Write its name in the table below.

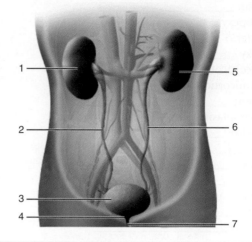

| kidney | ureter | urethra | sphincter | bladder |

	Name
1	
2	
3	
4	
5	
6	
7	

SELF-ASSESSMENT

Check (✓) what you learned. If you need more information or practice, refer to the relevant section in the chapter.

( ) I can name all the body systems.
( ) I can differentiate between the terms system, organ, and tissue.
( ) I can identify the organs of each system.
( ) I know the functions of each system.
( ) I can define and use the roots pertaining to each body system.
( ) I can analyze medical terms into their components.
( ) I can interpret the abbreviations pertaining to each system.
( ) I can use the new medical collocations and academic words properly.
( ) I can pronounce medical terms properly.
( ) I can skim and scan medical texts for main ideas and details.
( ) I can write a referral letter.
( ) I can spell and pronounce the new medical terms in the chapter.

Glossary

Medical Words	Meaning in English	Meaning in Arabic
abdominal	relating to the abdomen	بَطْنِيّ
abdominopelvic cavity	the space between the diaphragm and the groin	بَطْنِيّ، حَوضِيّ، جَوف
abduction	movement of a body part away from the median plane	تَبْعِيد
abnormal	not normal; differing in any way from the usual state	غَيرطَبيعِيّ؛غَيرْ سَوي
acetabulectomy	excision of the acetabulum (the cup-shaped cavity on the lateral surface of the hip bone)	اسْتِئصال الحَقّ
achromatopsia	a severe congenital deficiency in color perception, often associated with nystagmus and reduced visual acuity	عَمَى الألْوان
acrocyanosis	decrease in the amount of oxygen delivered to the extremities	زُراق الأطْراف
acromial	pertaining to the lateral extension of the spine of the scapula, forming the highest point of the shoulder	أخْرَمِيّ
adduct	to draw toward an axis or median line	يُقَرِّب
adduction	the act of adducting	تَقْرِيب
adenectomy	surgical excision of a gland	اسْتِئصال الغَدّة
adenocarcinoma	a malignant neoplasm of epithelial cells with a glandular or gland-like pattern	سَرَطانة غُدِّيّة
adenodynia	pain in a gland	ألَم غُدِّيّ
adenoid	pertaining to the pharyngeal tonsils	غُدّانِيّ
adenoidectomy	an operation for the removal of adenoid tissue from the nasopharynx	اسْتِئصال الغُدّانِيّات؛قَطْع الغُدّانِيّات
adenoma	a benign epithelial neoplasm in which the tumor cells form glands or gland-like structures	وَرَم غُدِّيّ؛غُدُّوم
adenomyosarcoma	a mixed mesodermal tumor containing striated muscle cells	ساركومة عَضَلِيّة غُدِّيّة؛غَرَن عَضَلِيّ غُدِّيّ
adenopathy	swelling or morbid enlargement of the lymph nodes	تَضَخُّم العَقد اللِّمفِيّة؛تَضَخُّم الغُدَد
adipocyte	a generic term for any fat-storing cell	خَلِيّة شَحمِيّة
adiposis	excessive local or general accumulation of fat in the body	شَحامة
adrenaline	hormone produced by medulla of the adrenal gland	أدْرينالين (أبِينفرِين)
adrenocorticotropic	pertaining to stimulation of the adrenal cortex	مُوَجِّه لِقِشْر الكُظْر (مُوَجِّه لِلْقِشْر)
adrenomegaly	an abnormal enlargement of one or both adrenal glands	ضَخامة الكُظْر
ageusia	absence or impairment of the sense of taste	فَقْد حاسّة الذَّوْق

Medical Words	Meaning in English	Meaning in Arabic
albinism	an inherited condition present at birth, characterized by a lack of pigment that normally gives color to the skin, hair, and eyes	مَهَق (برص)
albuminuria	presence of protein in urine	بِيلَة أَلْبومينِيّة
alveolar rhabdosarcoma	form of rhabdomyosarcoma occurring mainly in adolescents and young adults(a highly malignant neoplasm derived from striated muscle)	السّاركومة العَضَليّة المُخَطّطة السَّنْخِيّة
alveolitis	an inflammation of the alveoli, occurring either in the lungs or in the socket of a tooth	الْتِهاب الأَسْناخ
amblyopia	impaired vision with no discernible damage to the eye or optic nerve	غَمَش (ضَعْف الرُّؤْية دُون سَبَب عُضوي) واضح
amenorrhea	abnormal suppression or absence of menstruation	ضَهى؛ انْقِطاع الحَيض
amniocentesis	removal of some amniotic fluid by the insertion into the womb of a hollow needle	بَزْل السَّلى
amniorrhexis	rupture of the amnion	تَمَزُّق السَّلى
anal	relating to or located near the anus	شَرَجي
analgesia	insensibility to pain with no loss of consciousness	بُطْلان الأَلَم
anemia	a deficiency in the number of red blood cells or in their hemoglobin content	فَقَر الدَّم
anesthesia	local or general loss of bodily sensation	خَدَر (بُطْلان الحِسّ)
anesthetist	a person specially trained to administer anesthetics	تَقْني التَّخْدير؛ خَدّار
angiogram	an X-ray of one or more blood vessels following the injection of a radiopaque substance	صورة وعائِيّة
angiography	a method of obtaining an X-ray of blood vessels by injecting into them a substance that shows up as opaque on an X-ray picture	تَصْوير الأَوعِية
angiopoiesis	formation of blood or lymphatic vessels	تكَوُّن الأَوعِية
ankylosis	joint stiffening or fixation due to fibrous or bone union preventing articulation	قَسَط (رَكبة قسطاء: يَبِسَت وغَلَظت حتى لا تكاد تنفض من يبسها)
anoxia	a condition characterized by an absence of oxygen supply to an organ or a tissue	نَقْص الأَكْسجين؛عَوَز الأَكْسِجين
antebrachium	the segment of the upper limb between the elbow and the wrist	ساعِد
antenatal	occurring before birth	قَبْل الوِلادة
antepartum	occurring before childbirth	قَبْل الوَضْع
anterior	situated at or directed toward the front	أمامي
anthracosis	a chronic lung disease resulting from repeated inhalation of coal dust; inflammation of the lungs	سُحار فَحْمي
antibiotic	a substance, such as penicillin or erythromycin, produced by or derived from certain microorganisms that can destroy or inhibit the growth of other microorganisms	مُضادّ حيَوي؛صادّة
anxiolytic	a tranquilizer used to relieve anxiety and reduce tension and irritability	مُزيل القَلق
aortic stenosis	abnormal narrowing of the aortic valve	تَضيُّق الأَبْهَر

Medical Words	Meaning in English	Meaning in Arabic
aphakia	absence of the lens of an eye	انعدام العدسة
aphasia	a disorder of the central nervous system characterized by partial or total loss of the ability to communicate	حبسة
aphonia	loss of the voice resulting from disease, injury to the vocal cords	فقد الصوت
apnea	temporary absence or voluntary cessation of breathing	انقطاع النفس
appendectomy	surgical removal of the vermiform appendix	استئصال الزائدة
appendicitis	inflammation of the vermiform appendix	التهاب الزائدة
arteriolitis	inflammation of the wall of the arterioles	التهاب الشرينات
arteriomalacia	softening of the arteries	تلين الشرايين
arteriorrhaphy	suture of an artery	رفو الشريان
arteriosclerosis	hardening of the arteries	تصلب الشرايين تصلب شرياني
arteriospasm	spasm of an artery or arteries	تشنج الشريان
arteriostenosis	constriction of an artery	تضيق الشريان
arthralgia	pain in a joint	ألم مفصلي
arthritis	inflammation of a joint	التهاب المفصل
arthrodesis	surgical fusion of a joint	إيثاق المفصل
arthroscope	an endoscope for examining the internal anatomy of a joint	منظار المفصل
arthroscopy	examination of the interior of a joint with an arthroscope	تنظير المفصل
astroblast	a primordial cell developing into an astrocyte	أرومة نجمية
asynovia	absence or insufficiency of synovial secretion	ندرة الزليل
atherosclerosis	the build up of a waxy plaque on the inside of blood vessels	تصلب عصيدي
atriomegaly	abnormal enlargement of an atrium of the heart	ضخامة الأذين
audiometer	instrument used to measure the quality of a patient's hearing	مقياس السمع
audiometry	the measurement of hearing	قياس السمع
aural	pertaining to an aura	أذني
auriculocranial	pertaining to the auricle of the ear and the cranium	أذني قحفي
autopsy	an examination of the organs of a dead body to determine the cause of death	تشريح الجثة لتحديد سبب الوفاة
axillary	of or pertaining to the armpit	إبطي
bacteriostat	any agent that inhibits or retards bacterial multiplication	كابح الجراثيم
bacteriuria	the presence of bacteria in the urine	بيلة جرثومية
balanitis	an inflammation of the head and foreskin of the penis	التهاب الحشفة
basal-cell carcinoma	a locally invasive, rarely metastatic nevoid tumor of the epidermis	سرطان الخلايا القاعدية
bilateral	relating to both right and left sides of an area, organ, or organism	ثنائي الجانب
biliary	of or relating to bile, to the ducts that convey bile, or to the gall bladder	صفراوي
biologist	specialist in biology: the science of life and of living organisms	اختصاصي البيولوجيا

Medical Words	Meaning in English	Meaning in Arabic
biopsy	the removal and examination of a sample of tissue from a living body for diagnostic purposes	خَزْعَة؛ خَذْعَة؛ خِزْعَة
blepharoptosis	a drooping of the upper eyelid	إطراق
brachial	relating to the arm or to an arm-like part or structure	عَضُدِيّ
brachialgia	pain in the nerves of the upper arm	ألَم عَضُدِيّ
bradycardia	an abnormally low rate of heartbeat	بُطْءُ القَلْب (أقَل مِن 60 ضَرْبَة في الدَّقيقَة)
bradykinesia	abnormal slowness of physical movement	بُطْءُ الحَرَكَة
bradylalia	abnormally slow utterance due to a central nervous system lesion	ثِقَلُ النُّطْق
bronchiolectasis	dilatation of the bronchioles (small airways extending from the bronchi into the lobes of the lungs)	توَسُّعُ القُصَيْبات
bronchitis	chronic or acute inflammation of the mucous membrane of the bronchial tubes	التِهاب القَصَبات؛ التِهاب الشُّعَب الهَوائِيَّة
bronchoscope	an endoscope for inspecting the interior of the tracheobronchial tree	مِنْظار القَصَبات
bronchoscopy	inspection of the interior of the tracheobronchial tree through a bronchoscope	تَنْظير القَصَبات
bronchospasm	contraction of smooth muscles in the walls of the bronchi and bronchioles	تَشَنُّج قَصَبِيّ
buccoclusion	an occlusion in which the dental arch or group of teeth is buccal to the normal position	إطباق شِدْقِيّ
buccogingival	relating to the cheek and the gum	شِدْقِيّ لِثَوِيّ
bursitis	the painful inflammation of the bursa (a pad-like sac found in areas subject to friction)	التِهاب الجِراب
calcaneodynia	pain in the heel	ألَم العَقِب
calcipenia	a deficiency of calcium in the body tissues and fluids	قِلَّة الكالْسِيُوم
calicectomy	excision of a calix of the kidney	اسْتِئْصال الكَأْس
calioplasty	surgical reconstruction of a calix (a cuplike organ or cavity)	جِراحَة الكَأْس
calorimeter	an instrument for measuring the amount of heat produced in any system or organism	مِقْياس الكالوري؛ مِكْلار
capnogram	a continuous record of the carbon dioxide content of expired air	تَصْوير الكَبِد الكَرْبونِيّ
carcinogen	any cancer-producing substance or organism	مُسَرْطِن
carcinoma	an invasive malignant tumor derived from epithelial tissue that tends to metastasize to other areas of the body	سَرَطانَة
cardiac	pertaining to the heart	قَلْبِيّ
cardiologist	a physician skilled in the diagnosis and treatment of heart disease	طَبيب القَلْب
cardiology	study of the heart and its functions	طِبُّ القَلْب
cardiomegaly	enlargement of the heart	تَضَخُّم القَلْب
cardiomyopathy	a chronic disease of the heart muscle	اعْتِلال عَضَلَة القَلْب
cardionecrosis	death of heart tissue	تَخَرُّ القَلْب
cardiopathy	any disorder or disease of the heart	اعْتِلال القَلْب
cardiovascular	pertaining to the heart and blood vessels	قَلْبِيّ وِعائيّ

Medical Words	Meaning in English	Meaning in Arabic
carpoptosis	paralysis of the extensors of the wrist and fingers	تَدَلّي الرُّسْغ
caudal	pertaining to the tail	ذَنَبِيّ
cecoptosis	falling displacement of the cecum (the first part of the large intestine)	رَفْو الأعْوَر
celiac	relating to the abdominal cavity	بَطْنيّ
celioma	a tumor of the abdomen	وَرَم بَطْنيّ
celioscopy	examination or treatment of the interior of the abdomen	تَنْظيرُ البَطْن
cephalad	toward the head	رَأْسِيّا (باتجاه الرأس)
cephaledema	edema of the head	وَذَمَة الرَّأْس
cephalic	pertaining to the head	رَأْسِيّ
cerebral	pertaining to the cerebrum or the largest part of the brain	مُخّيّ
cerebrosclerosis	morbid hardening of the substance of the cerebrum	تَصَلُّب المُخّ
cerebrovascular	pertaining to the blood vessels of the cerebrum or brain	دِماغِيّ وِعائِيّ
cerebrum	the largest portion of the brain	اكبر جزء في المُخّ
ceruminolytic	one of several substances instilled into the external auditory canal to soften wax	حالّ الصِّمْلاخ
cervical	pertaining to the neck or the uterine cervix	رَقَبيّ
cervical carcinoma	a disease in which the cells of the cervix become abnormal and start to grow uncontrollably, forming tumors	قَبصَريّة عَنْق الرَّحِم (قَبصَريّة القِطعَة) السُّفْلِيّة
cervicitis	an inflammation of the cervix	الْتِهاب عَنْق الرَّحِم
cheiloplasty	plastic surgery of the lip	رَأْب الشَّفَة
chemotherapy	treatment of cancer with anticancer drugs	مُعالَجَة كيميائِيّة
chloropia	a sign of digitalis toxicity in which viewed objects appear green	اخْضِرار الرُّؤْيَة
cholangioma	a neoplasm of bile duct origin, especially within the liver; may be either benign or malignant	وَرَم الأقْنِيَة الصَّفْراوِيَة
cholangiosarcoma	sarcoma of bile duct origin	غَعْرَ القَناة الصَّفْراوِيَة
cholecystectomy	the surgical removal of the gallbladder	اسْتِئْصال المَرارَة
cholecystogram	a radiograph of the gallbladder	صورَة المَرارَة
choledochotomy	incision into the common bile duct	بَضْع قَناة الصَّفْراء
cholestasis	stoppage or suppression of bile flow	رُكود صَفْراوِيّ
chondrocarcinoma	a malignant epithelial tumor in which cartilaginous metaplasia is present	سَرَطانَة غُضْروفِيّة
chondrosarcoma	a malignant tumor derived from cartilage cells or their precursors	ساركومة غُضْروفِيّة
chronic	lasting for a long period of time or marked by frequent recurrence	مُزْمِن
chronotropic	affecting the time or rate	مُؤَثّر على الميقاتِيّة
cirrhosis	a chronic degenerative disease in which normal liver cells are damaged and are then replaced by scar tissue	تَشَمّع؛ تَلَيُّف
clavicular	pertaining to the clavicle (collarbone)	تَرْقُوِي
clitorectomy	excision of the clitoris (the small, elongated, erectile body in the female)	اسْتِئْصال البَظْر

Medical Words	Meaning in English	Meaning in Arabic
coccygeal	pertaining to or located in the region of the coccyx	عُصْعُصِيّ
coccyx (tailbone)	the small bone at the end of the vertebral column in humans, formed by the fusion of four rudimentary vertebrae	عُصْعُص
cochleitis	inflammation of the cochlea (a spiral tube shaped like a snail shell, forming part of the inner ear)	التهاب القوقعة
colectomy	excision of a segment or of the entire colon	استئصال القولون
colocolostomy	surgical formation of an anastomosis between two portions of the colon	مُفاغرة قولونية قولونية
colonoscopy	visual examination of the inner surface of the colon by means of a colonoscope	تنظير القولون
colorectal carcinoma	a malignant epithelial tumor arising from the colonic or rectal mucosa	سرطانة القولون المُستقيم
colostomy	the surgical creation of an opening between the colon and the body surface	فغْر القولون
colposcopy	examination of the vaginal and cervical epithelia by means of a colposcope	تنظير المهبل
colpostenosis	narrowing of the lumen of the vagina	تضيق المهبل
condylectomy	excision of a condyle (a rounded projection on a bone, usually for articulation with another bone)	استئصال اللُقمة
conjunctivoplasty	plastic repair of the conjunctiva (the delicate membrane lining the eyelids)	رأب المُلتحمة
coreoplasty	any plastic operation on the pupil	رأب الفَرجية
corneoblepharon	adhesion of the eyelid margin to the cornea	التصاق جفْني قرنوي
coronary	pertaining to the heart	تاجي
corticospinal	pertaining to or connecting the cerebral cortex and spinal cord	قشري نُخاعي
cranial	relating to the cranium or head	قحْفي
craniomalacia	abnormal softness of the bones of the skull	تليُّن القحْف
craniotomy	surgical removal of part of the skull to expose the brain	حجّ القحْف
cryotherapy	the use of cold in the treatment of disease	مُعالجة بالبرد
cutaneous	pertaining to the skin	جلْدي
cyanophil	a cell or element that is differentially colored blue by a staining procedure	أليف الأزرق
cyclodialysis	creation of a communication between the anterior chamber of the eye and the suprachoroidal space in glaucoma	فصْل الجسم الهدبي
cystitis	inflammation of the urinary bladder	التهاب المثانة
cystoscopy	examination of the bladder by means of a cystoscope	تنظير المثانة
cystotomy	incision or puncture into urinary bladder	بضْع المثانة
cytologist	a biologist who specializes in the study of cells	اختصاصي السيتولوجيا
cytopenia	deficiency in numbers of any of the blood cell elements	قلّة الكُريات
dacryorrhea	excessive flow of tears	دُماع
dactylitis	inflammation of one or more fingers	التهاب الإصبع
dactylospasm	spasmodic contraction of the fingers or toes	تشنُّج الأصابع

Medical Words	Meaning in English	Meaning in Arabic
decubitus position	a position used in producing a radiograph of the chest or abdomen of a patient who is lying down, with the central ray horizontal	وَضْعِيّةُ الاسْتِلْقاء
deep (internal)	positioned internally at or toward the center	عَميق داخِلي
dentist	a person who is trained and licensed to practice dentistry	طَبيبُ الأسْنان
dermal	pertaining to the skin	جِلْدي
dermatitis	inflammation of the skin	الْتِهابُ الجِلْد
dermatologist	a physician specializing in the skin and its properties of health and disease	طَبيبُ الجِلْد
dermatology	the medical specialty concerned with the diagnosis and treatment of skin diseases	طِبُّ الجِلْد
dermatosis	any noninflammatory disorder of the skin	مرض جلدي
diagnosis	determination of the nature of a cause of a disease	تَشْخيص
diameter	the distance measured along such a line	قُطْر
diarrhea	an abnormally frequent discharge of semisolid or fluid fecal matter from the bowel	إسْهال
digestive	pertaining to digestion (the process in the alimentary canal by which food is broken up physically and chemically	هَضْمي
diplopia	double vision: a condition whereby a single object appears as two objects	شَفَع (ازْدِواجُ الرُّؤْية)
distal	remote; farther from any point of reference	قاصٍ
dorsal (posterior)	pertaining to the back	ظَهْراني، خَلْفي
dorsal cavity	composed of the cranial and spinal cavities	التجويف الخلفي
dorsal recumbent	lying on the back, as in a supine position	وَضْعِيّةُ الاسْتِلْقاء الظَّهْري
duodenojejunostomy	anastomosis of the duodenum to the jejunum)the first and second part of the small intestine)	مُفاغَرَةٌ إثْناعَشَرِيّةٌ صائِمِيّة
duodenoscope	an endoscope for examining the duodenum	مِنْظار الإثْناعَشَري
duodenostomy	surgical formation of a permanent opening into the duodenum	بَضْعُ الإثْناعَشَري
duodenum	the first or proximal portion of the small intestine	الإثْناعَشَري
dysentery	a disease marked by frequent watery stools, often with blood and mucus	زُحار
dysesthesia	impairment of any sense, especially of the sense of touch	ضَعْفُ الحِسّ
dyslexia	inability to read, spell, and write words	خَلَلُ القِراءة
dysmenorrheal	the occurrence of painful cramps during menstruation	عَسيرةُ الطَّمْث
dyspepsia	impairment of the power or function of digestion	عُسْرُ الهَضْم
dysphagia	difficulty or inability to swallow	عُسْرُ البَلْع
dysplasia	alteration in size, shape, and organization of adult cells	خَلَلُ التَّنَسُّج، نَدَن
dyspnea	difficulty in breathing	ضيقُ النَّفَس، زُلّة
dystocia	abnormal labor or childbirth	عُسْرُ الولادة
dysuria	painful or difficult urination	عُسْرُ التَّبَوُّل
echography	the location, measurement, or delineation of deep structures by measuring the reflection or transmission of high-frequency or ultrasonic waves	تَخْطيطُ الصَّدى

Medical Words	Meaning in English	Meaning in Arabic
edentulous	without teeth	عديم الأَسْنان
electromyography	an electrical recording of muscle activity that aids in the diagnosis of neuromuscular disease	مُخَطِّط كَهْرَبِيّة للعضل
electrocardiogram	a record of the electrical activity of the heart	مُخَطِّط كَهْرَبِيّة القلب
electrocardiograph	an instrument for recording the potential of the electrical currents that traverse the heart	مِخْطاط كَهْرَبِيّة القلب
electrocardiography	a method of recording electrical activity generated by the heart muscle	مِخْطاط كَهْرَبِيّة القلب
electrocraniography	a method of recording electrical activity generated by the skull	توصيف كهربية القَحْف
electroencephalogram	a graphic record of the electrical activity of the brain as recorded by an electroencephalograph	مُخَطِّط كَهْرَبِيّة الدّماغ
electroencephalography	a neurological test that uses an electronic monitoring device to measure and record electrical activity in the brain	تخطيط كَهْرَبِيّة الدّماغ
electrophoresis	the movement of particles in an electric field toward a node or cathode	رَحَلان كَهْرَبِيّ
embolectomy	surgical removal of an embolus (a clot or other plug)	استئصال الصِّمَّة
embryonic	pertaining to, or in the condition of an embryo	مُضْغِيّ
emphysema	a pathologic accumulation of air in tissues or organs	نَفَاخ
encephalitis	an inflammation of the brain	التهاب الدّماغ
endocrine	the internal or hormonal secretion of a ductless gland	صمّاوي
endocrine glands	glands that have no ducts, their secretions being absorbed directly into the blood	الغُدَد الصّمّاء
endocrinologist	a physician who specializes in the endocrine system and its disorders	اختصاصيّ الغُدَد الصُّمّ
endocrinology	a medical specialty concerned with the diagnosis and treatment of disorders of the endocrine system	عِلْم الغُدَد الصُّمّ
endometrium	the mucous membrane lining the uterus	بِطانة الرَّحِم
endoscope	an instrument for examining the interior of a hollow viscus	مِنْظار داخِلي
epididymotomy	incision into the epididymis (an elongated, cord-like structure along the posterior border of the testis)	بَضْع البَرْبَخ
epiglottitis	inflammation of the epiglottis (the lid-like cartilaginous structure overhanging the entrance to the larynx)	التهاب لِسان المِزْمار
epiphysis	a part of a long bone developed from a secondary center of ossification	الكردوس
episiotomy	surgical incision of the perineum during childbirth to facilitate delivery	بَضْع الفَرْج
epithelial	pertaining to or composed of epithelium (lining of internal organs and outer layer of skin cells)	ظهاري
ergograph	an instrument for measuring work done in muscular action	مِخْطاط العَمَل
ergometry	the study of physical work activity	قِياس الدّينَمِيّة
erythema	redness of the skin	حُمامى/ التهاب احمراري للجلد
erythroblastosis	the presence of erythroblasts in considerable numbers in the blood	كَثْرة أرُومات الحَمْر

Medical Words	Meaning in English	Meaning in Arabic
erythrocyte	a mature red blood cell	كُرَيّة حَمْراء
erythrocytopenia	deficiency in the number of red blood cells	قَلّة الكُرَيّات الحَمْر
erythropoiesis	the formation of red blood cells	تَكَوُّن الكُرَيّات الحَمْر
esophageal	pertaining to the esophagus (the muscular tube by which food passes from the pharynx to the stomach)	مَريئي
esophageal osteosarcoma	cancerous tumor of the esophagus	ساركومة عَظْمِيّة المَريئ
esophagitis	inflammation of the esophagus	التِهاب المَريء
esophagoscopy	visual examination of the esophagus	تَنْظير المَريء
etiology	the science dealing with causes of disease	السَّبَبِيّات/ عِلم أسباب الأمراض
eucapnia	a state in which the arterial carbon dioxide pressure is optimal	سَوائِيّة ثاني أُكْسيد الكَرْبون في الدَّم
euphoria	a feeling of well-being	شَمَق (الشَّمَق: النَّشاط ومَرَح الجنون)
eupnea	normal respiration	سَوائِيّة التَّنَفُّس
euthanasia	an easy or painless death	قَتْل المَرْحَمة (تيسير الموت في الأمراض التي لايُرجى شفاؤها)
eversion	a turning inside out; a turning outward	انْقِلاب للخارج
Ewing sarcoma	a malignant tumor that develops from bone marrow, usually in long bones or the pelvis	ساركومة يوينْغ (في العظام)
exocrine glands	mucous glands which secrete on to a surface	غُدَد خارجِيّة الإفْراز
extrapulmonary	outside or having no relation to the lungs	خارج الرِّئة
fasciodesis	surgical attachment of a fascia to another fascia or a tendon	تَثْبيت اللَّفافة (بالعَظْم)
femoral	pertaining to the femur or to the thigh	فَخْذي
fetometry	measurement of the fetus, especially of its head	قِياس الجَنين
fibroma	a benign neoplasm derived from fibrous connective tissue	وَرَم لِيفي
fibrosarcoma	a malignant neoplasm derived from deep fibrous tissue	ساركومة لِيفِيّة
fibulocalcaneal	relating to the fibula (the lateral and smaller of the two bones of the lower leg) and the calcaneus (the largest of the tarsal bones)	شَظَوي عَقِبي
foramen	a natural opening or passage, especially one into or through a bone	ثُقوب
Fowler's position	the posture assumed by the patient when the head of the bed is raised 90 degrees and his or her knees are elevated slightly	وَضْعِيّة فاولِر (وَضعية المريض في السرير برفع رأسه وركبتيه للأعلى)
fructose	a sugar that occurs naturally in fruits and honey	فِرِكْتوز
galactopoiesis	secretion and continued production of milk by the mammary glands	تَكْوين اللَّبَن
ganglionectomy	excision of a ganglion (group of nerve cells)	اسْتِئْصال العُقْدة
gastrectasia	dilation of the stomach	تَوَسُّع المَعِدة
gastric	pertaining to the stomach	مَعِدي
gastritis	inflammation, especially mucosal, of the stomach	التِهاب المَعِدة
gastrocele	hernial protrusion of the stomach	قَيْلة مَعِدِيّة
gastroenteritis	inflammation of the stomach and intestine	التِهاب المَعِدة والأمْعاء

Medical Words	Meaning in English	Meaning in Arabic
gastroenterologist	physician who specializes in diseases affecting the GI tract	طبيب الجهاز الهضمي
gastroenterology	the study of the stomach and intestine and their diseases	طب الجهاز الهضمي
gastrojejunostomy	surgical anastomosis of the stomach to the jejunum (the second part of the small intestine)	مُفاغرة معديّة صائميّة
gastropexy	surgical fixation of the stomach	تثبيت المَعِدة
gastroscopy	examination of the mucosal surface of the stomach by an upper GI endoscope	تنظير المَعِدة
geriatrics	the branch of medicine concerned with the health care of the elderly	طب الشُيوخ
gingivitis	inflammation of the gingiva (the part of the oral mucosa covering the tooth-bearing border of the jaw)	التهاب اللّثة
glioma	a tumor composed of neuroglia in any of its states of development	ورم دبقي
glomerulitis	inflammation of the glomeruli of the kidney	التهاب الكُبَيبات
glossoplegia	paralysis of the tongue	شلَل اللّسان
glucogenesis	formation of glucose	تكوُن الغلوكوز
glycolysis	the pathway in which a cell breaks down glucose into energy	تحلُل السكُر
gnathic	pertaining to the jaw or cheeks	فكّي
gonadotropin	a hormone that stimulates the growth and activity of the gonads (the sex glands)	موَجهة الغدد التناسليّة
gynecologist	a physician who specializes in the medical care of conditions unique to women	طبيب النسائيّات
gynecology	the medical specialty concerned with diseases of the female genital tract	طب النساء ؛ النسائيّات
hemangioma	a benign tumor consisting of a mass of blood vessels	ورم وعائي
hematemesis	vomiting of blood	قيء الدّم
hematocrit	the percentage by volume of packed red blood cells in a given sample of blood after centrifugation	الهيماتوكريت (حجم الكُريّات الحمْر) المكدوسة
hematologist	specialist in the composition and analysis of blood	اختصاصي الدّمويّات
hematoma	a localized swelling filled with blood resulting from a break in a blood vessel	ورم دَموي
hematorrhagia	bursting forth of blood	انْتزاف (نزف غزير)
hematuria	the presence of blood in the urine	بيلة دَمويّة
hemigastrectomy	surgical removal of one half of the stomach	استئصال المَعِدة الجزئي
hemiplegia	paralysis of one side of the body	فالج ؛ شلَل نصفي
hemoglobin	the protein in the red blood cells	هيموغلوبين ؛ خضاب الدّم
hemolysis	destruction or dissolution of red blood cells, with subsequent release of hemoglobin	حلُ الدّم
hemopoiesis	the formation of blood	تكوُن الدّم
hemorrhage	excessive discharge of blood from the blood vessels; profuse bleeding	نزف
hepatectomy	surgical removal of all or part of the liver	استئصال الكبد
hepatitis	inflammation of the liver	التهاب الكبد

Medical Words	Meaning in English	Meaning in Arabic
hepatohemia	rarely used term for congestion of the liver	احتِقانُ الكَبِد
hepatoma	a tumor of the liver	وَرَمٌ كَبِديّ
hepatomegaly	enlargement of the liver	تَضَخُّم الكَبِد
hepatorrhexis	rupture of the liver	تَمَزُّقُ الكَبِد
herniotomy	surgical division of the constriction or strangulation of a hernia	بَضْعُ الفَتْق
heterochromic	pertaining to heterochromia (a difference in coloration in two structures that are normally alike in color)	مُغايِرُ اللَّون
hidradenitis	inflammation of the sweat glands	الْتِهاب الغُدَد العَرَقِيَّة
histology	the science of diseased tissues	الهِيستولوجيا؛عِلْمُ الأَنْسِجَة
humeroscapular	pertaining to the humerus (the bone of the upper arm) and scapula (the flat triangular bone in the back of the shoulder)	عَضُدِيٌّ كَتِفِيّ
hydrocele	a collection of serous fluid in a sacculated cavity	أُدْرة (قِيلَةٌ مائِيَّة)
hyperglycemia	an abnormally high concentration of glucose in the circulating blood	فَرْطُ سُكَّرِ الدَّم
hypertension	abnormally elevated arterial blood pressure	فَرْطُ الضَّغْط
hypnosis	an altered state of consciousness	تَنْويم
hypochondriac	pertaining to the regions of the upper abdomen beneath the lower ribs	مَراقِيّ
hypogastric	pertaining to the hypogastrium, the lower abdominal region	خَثَلِيّ
hypoglycemia	an abnormally low level of glucose in the blood	نَقْصُ سُكَّرِ الدَّم
hypophyseal	pertaining to the pituitary gland	نُخامِيّ
hypoproteinemia	deficiency of protein in the blood	نَقْصُ بروتين الدَّم
hypotension	abnormally low arterial blood pressure	نَقْصُ الضَّغْط
hypothyroidism	insufficient production of thyroid hormones	قُصورُ الدَّرَقِيَّة
hysterectomy	the surgical removal of the uterus	اسْتِئصال الرَّحِم
ichthyosis	congenital dermatological (skin) disease that is represented by thick, scaly skin	سَمَاك
idiopathic	self-originated; occurring without known cause	مَجْهولُ السَّبَب
ileitis	inflammation of the ileum (the last part of the small intestine)	الْتِهاب اللَّفائِفيّ
iliac	pertaining to the hip bone	حَرْقَفيّ
ilium	the lateral, flaring portion of the hip bone	الحَرْقَفَة
immunization	a process or procedure that protects the body against an infectious disease	تَمْنيع ؛ تَحْصين
inferior (caudal)	nearer the soles of the feet	السُّفْلِيّ / ذَنَبيّ
inguinal	pertaining to the groin (the junctional region between the abdomen and thigh)	أُرْبِيّ
insomnia	inability to sleep	أَرَق
insular	a pyramid-shaped area of the brain within each cerebral hemisphere beneath parts of the frontal and temporal lobes; also called: island of Reil	جَزيرِيّ
integumentary	relating to the integument (skin)	جِلْدِيّ

Medical Words	Meaning in English	Meaning in Arabic
interatrial	between the atria of the heart	بين الأُذَينَين
intermediate	organ between right and left (or lateral and medial) structures	مُتَوَسِّط
intervertebral	between two vertebrae	بين الفِقْرَتين
intravenous	within a vein	داخِل الوَرِيد،وَرِيدي
intraventricular	within a ventricle of the brain or heart	داخِل البَطين
inversion	a turning inward, inside out, or other reversal of the normal relation of a part	انقِلاب
iridocele	hernial protrusion of part of the iris through the cornea	قَيلَة قَزَحِيَّة
iridopupillary	pertaining to the iris and pupil of the eye	قَزَحيّ حَدَقي
ischemia	an insufficient supply of blood to an organ	إقفار،نَقص التَرْوِية
ischiodynia	pain in the ischium (the inferior, dorsal portion of the hip bone)	ألَم الإسْك
jaundice	yellowish discoloration of the whites of the eyes, skin, and mucous membranes	يَرَقان
jejunoileostomy	surgical creation of an anastomosis between the proximal jejunum and the terminal ileum	مُفاغَرة صائِمِيَّة لَفائِفِيَّة
karyoclasis	fragmentation of the nucleus	تَفَتُّت النَواة
karyolysis	destruction of the nucleus of a cell	انحِلال النَواة
keratolysis	loosening or separation of the horny layer of the epidermis	انحِلال الطَبَقة القَرنِيَّة
kinesis	movement or activity of an organism in response to a stimulus such as light	حَرَكة ؛ تَحَرُّك
kinesitherapy	treatment of disease by movements or exercise	مُعالَجة بالحَرَكة
knee-chest position	a prone posture resting on the knees and upper part of the chest	وَضْعِيَّة التَجَبِّية
kyphosis	the extreme curvature of the upper back	الحَداب
labium	any lip-shaped structure	الشُِفَة
labyrinthitis	an inflammation of the inner ear	التِهاب التِيه
lacrimotomy	incision of the lacrimal gland, duct, or sac	بَضْع المَدامِع
lactogenesis	the production of milk	إفْراز اللَبَن
laminectomy	excision of the posterior arch of a vertebra	استِئصال الصَفيحة الفِقَرِية
laparoscope	an endoscope for examining the peritoneal cavity	مِنْظار البَطْن (مِنْظار الصِفاق)
laparoscopy	examination of the peritoneal cavity by means of the laparoscope	تَنْظير البَطْن (تَنْظير الصِفاق)
laparotomy	incision through the abdominal wall	بَضْع البَطْن ؛ فَتْح البَطْن
laryngectomy	the partial or complete surgical removal of the larynx (voice box)	استِئصال الحَنْجَرة
laryngoscope	a diagnostic instrument that is used to examine the interior of the larynx	مِنْظار الحَنْجَرة
laryngoscopy	examination of the larynx by means of a laryngoscope	تَنْظير الحَنْجَرة
lateral	pertaining to a side	جانبي
left hypochondriac	pertaining to the left regions of the upper abdomen beneath the lower ribs and lateral to the epigastric region	مَراقي الأيسَر

Medical Words	Meaning in English	Meaning in Arabic
left iliac (inguinal)	pertaining to the left hip bone	الحرقفي الأيسر
left lateral recumbent	a position in which the patient lies on the left side with the upper knee and thigh drawn upward	الاستلقاء على الجانب الأيسر
left lower quadrant or LLQ	the region of the body that contains the left ovary and adnexae and rectosigmoid colon	الربع السفلي الأيسر
left lumbar	relating to the left loins, or the part of the back and sides between the ribs and the pelvis	قطني الأيسر
left upper quadrant or LUQ	the left region of the body containing the stomach, spleen and tail of pancreas	الربع العلوي الأيسر
leiomyoma	a benign neoplasm derived from smooth (nonstriated) muscle	وَرَم عَضَلِيّ أَمْلَس
lentiform	lens shaped	عَدَسِيّ الشَكْل
leptomeningopathy	any disease of the leptomeninges (the arachnoid membrane and the pia mater)	اعْتِلال السَّحايا الرَّقيقة
leukapheresis	the selective removal of leukocytes from withdrawn blood	فَصادة الكُرَيّات البيض
leukemia	malignant disease of the blood-forming organs	سرطان الدم
leukocyte	white blood cell that protects the body against infection and fight infection when it occurs	كُرَيّة بيضاء
leukocytosis	a condition characterized by an elevated number of white cells in the blood	كَثرة الكُرَيّات البيض
leukopenia	an abnormally low number of leukocytes in the circulating blood	قِلّة الكُرَيّات البيض
leukoplakia	an abnormal condition characterized by white spots or patches on mucous membranes of the mouth	طُلوان
ligamentous	relating to or of the form or structure of a ligament	رباطي
lingual	pertaining to the tongue	لِساني
lipocele	a hernia containing only fat within the hernial sac	قيلة شَحْمِيّة
lipoma	a benign fatty tumor usually composed of mature fat cells	وَرَم شَحْمي
liposarcoma	a very rare malignant tumor of fatty tissue	ساركومة شَحْمِيّة
lithotomy position	a supine position in which the hips and knees are fully flexed with the legs spread apart and raised and the feet resting in straps	وضعية استلقاء ظهرية عجزية
lithotripsy	the crushing of a stone in the renal pelvis, calyces, ureter, or bladder	تَفْتيت الحَصاة
lobectomy	surgical excision of a lobe, as of the lung, brain, liver, or thyroid	اسْتِئصال الفَص
lordosis	the anterior concavity in the curvature of the lumbar and cervical spine	قَعَس / البزخ إنحناء العمود الفقري
lumbar	relating to the loins, or the part of the back and sides between the ribs and the pelvis	قَطني
lymphadenocele	a cyst of a lymph node	قيلة العُقْدة اللِّمْفِيّة
lymphadenopathy	any disease process affecting a lymph node or lymph nodes	تَضَخُّم العُقَد اللِّمْفِيّة
lymphangiofibroma	a term that dignifies a common lymphangioma with prominent fibrosis	وَرَم وعائي لِمْفي لِيفي

Medical Words	Meaning in English	Meaning in Arabic
lymphangitis	inflammation of a lymphatic vessel	الْتِهاب الأوْعِية اللّمْفِية
lymphatic	pertaining to lymph or to a lymphatic vessel	لِمْفاوِي
lymphocyte	a type of white blood cell that is important in the formation of antibodies	اللّمْفاوِية
lymphocytic	pertaining to lymphocytes	لِمْفاوِي
lymphoma	malignant tumors that arise from the lymphocytic cells of the immune system	وَرَم لِمْفي
lymphosarcoma	malignant neoplastic disorders of lymphoid tissue	ساركُومة لِمْفِية
macroscopic	of a size visible with the unaided eye or without the use of a microscope	عِياني
mammary	relating to the breasts	ثَدْيي
mammogram	a radiograph of the breast	صورة الثَّدْي الشُّعاعِية
mammography	the study of the breast using X-ray	تَصْوير الثَّدْي الشُّعاعي
mammoplasty	plastic surgery of the breast	رَأْب الثَّدْي
mastectomy	the surgical removal of the breast	اسْتِئْصال الثَّدْي
mastitis	inflammation of a mammary gland or udder	الْتِهاب الثَّدْي
mastoiditis	an infection of the spaces within the mastoid bone (the prominent bone behind the ear)	الْتِهاب الخَشّاء
maxillofacial	pertaining to the jaws and face	فَكّ-عُلْوي وَجْهي
meatotomy	a form of penile modification in which the underside of the glans is split	بَضْع الصِّماخ
medial	toward the center	إنْسي
mediastinitis	inflammation of the tissues in the mid-chest	الْتِهاب المَنْصِف
mediastinum	an undelineated group of structures in the thorax	المَنْصِف الأمامي
medullary	the inner core of certain organs or body structures	نُخاعي
megacolon	an abnormal enlargement of the colon	تَضَخُّم القَوْلُون
megalomania	a mental illness characterized by delusions of grandeur, power, and wealth	هَوَس العَظَمة
melanocyte	an epidermal cell capable of synthesizing melanin	خَلِية مِيلانِينية
melanoma	malignant tumor arising from a melanocyte and occurring most commonly in the skin	وَرَم مِيلانيني
meningitis	inflammation of the membranes that surround the brain or spinal cord	الْتِهاب السَّحايا السَّرَطاني
meningococci	the bacteria that cause cerebrospinal meningitis	المُكَوَّرات السَّحائِية
menopause	the permanent cessation of menstruation	إياس
menorrhagia	excessive bleeding during menstruation	غَزارة الطَّمْث
menorrhea	menstrual flow	الحَيْض
menostasis	stoppage of the menses	ضَهَى ؛ انْعِدام الحَيْض
metacarpectomy	surgical excision of one or all of the metacarpals of the hand	اسْتِئْصال السَّنَع
metric	pertaining to measures or measurement	مِتْري
metropathy	any disease of the uterus	اعْتِلال الرَّحِم
microscope	an instrument used to obtain an enlarged image of small objects	مِجْهَر

Medical Words	Meaning in English	Meaning in Arabic
microtome	an instrument for making thin sections for microscopic study	مِشراحٌ دَقيقٌ
modified Trendelenburg	a supine position in which the feet are higher than the head; used in patients who become acutely hypotensive	وضعِيَةُ ترِنَد إِنبورغ (وضعية استلقائية مائلة) مع تدلي الرأس
morphosis	the process of formation of a part or organ	التَشكُّلُ العُضوِيّ
multicellular	composed of many cells	مُتعدِّدُ الخَلايا
muscular	pertaining to a muscle	عَضَلِيّ
musculoskeletal	pertaining to muscle and skeleton	عَضَلِيّ هَيكَلِيّ
myalgia	muscular pain	ألَمٌ عَضَلِيّ
mycology	the study of fungi and fungal diseases	علْمُ الفُطرِيّات
myelogenous	produced in the bone marrow	نِقيي المَنشأ
myelitis	inflammation of the spinal cord or bone marrow	التهابُ النُخاع
myelogram	an X-ray of the spinal cord	صورةُ النُخاع
myocardial	pertaining to the muscular tissue of the heart	متعلق بعَضَلِ القَلب
myolysis	disintegration or degeneration of muscle tissue	تحلُّلُ العَضَل
myoma	a benign neoplasm of muscular tissue	ورمٌ عَضَلِيّ أملس
myoparesis	slight muscle paralysis	خَزَلُ العَضَلَة
myorrhexis	rupture of a muscle	تمَزُّقٌ عَضَلِيّ
myosarcoma	a malignant neoplasm derived from muscular tissue	ساركومةٌ عَضَلِيّةٌ
myositis	inflammation of a voluntary muscle	التهابُ العَضَل
myringotomy	incision of the tympanic membrane	بَضعُ الطَّبلَة
narcolepsy	a disorder featuring an overwhelming tendency to fall asleep	تَغفيق
narcosis	a condition of deep stupor or unconsciousness	تخَدُّر
nasal	pertaining to the nose	أنفي
necrosis	death of cells through injury or disease	تنَخُّر
neoplastic	pertaining to neoplasia or neoplasm (any new and abnormal growth)	ورَمِيّ
nephrectomy	the surgical procedure of removing a kidney	استِئصالُ الكُلية
nephrologist	a doctor who specializes in the diseases and disorders of the kidneys	طبيبُ الكُلى
nephroma	a tumor of kidney tissue	ورَمٌ كُلوِيّ
nephropathy	any disease of the kidneys	اعتِلالُ الكُلية
nephrotoxin	substance that is poisonous to the kidneys	سمٌّ كُلوِيّ
nervous	relating to a nerve or the nerves	عَصبِيّ
neuralgia	abnormal condition that affects the nervous system	ألَمٌ عَصبِيّ
neurasthenia	an ill-defined condition, commonly accompanying or following depression, characterized by vague fatigue believed to be brought on by psychological factors	وهَنٌ عَصبِيّ
neuromimetic	relating to the action of a drug that mimics the response of an effector organ to nerve impulses	محاكي الاستجابة العصبية
neuritis	inflammation of a nerve	التهابُ العَصَب؛ التِهابٌ عَصبِيّ
neurology	the branch of medicine that deals with the nervous system	طبُّ الأعصاب؛ طبُّ الجِهاز العصَبِيّ

Medical Words	Meaning in English	Meaning in Arabic
neuroplasty	plastic repair of a nerve	رَأبُ العَصَب
noctalbuminuria	the excretion of protein into the urine	بيلةُ ألبُومينيةٌ ليليّة
nocturia	excessive urination at night	بَوالٌ ليلي
normocapnia	a state in which the arterial carbon dioxide pressure is normal	سواءيّةُ ثُنائي أُكسيد كربون الدّم
obstetrics	the specialty of medicine concerned with the care of women during pregnancy	طبُّ التّوليد
ocular	pertaining to the eye	العَينيّة (في المِجهَر)/ عَيني
oncologist	a physician who specializes in the study and treatment of neoplastic diseases	اختِصاصي الأورام
onychomalacia	abnormal softness of the nails	تليُنُ الظُفر
oocyte	an immature ovum	الخَليّةُ البيضيّة
oophorectomy	the surgical removal of one or both ovaries	استِئصال المَبيض
oophoritis	inflammation of an ovary	التِهاب المَبيض
ophthalmologist	a physician who specializes in the treatment of the eye	طبيب العُيون
ophthalmoscope	an instrument for examining the interior of the eye	مِنظار العَين
optician	one that makes lenses and eyeglasses	نظاراتي ؛ اختِصاصي البَصريّات
optometer	an instrument for determining the refraction of the eye	مِقياس البَصَر
oral	relating to the mouth	فمَوي
orchialgia	pain in the testis	ألمُ الخُصيَة
orchidectomy	removal of one or both testes	استِئصال الخُصيَة
orchiopexy	surgical treatment of an undescended testicle	تثبيت الخُصيَة
orchitis	an inflammation of the testis	التِهاب الخُصيَة
oropharynx	the part of the pharynx between the soft palate and the upper edge of the epiglottis	البُلعوم الفمَوي (الجزءُ الفمَوي من البُلعوم)
orthodontics	that branch of dentistry concerned with the correction and prevention of irregularities and malocclusion of the teeth	تقويم الأسنان
orthopedics	the branch of medicine that deals with the prevention or correction of injuries or disorders of the skeletal system and associated muscles, joints, and ligaments	جراحةُ العِظام
orthopedist	a physician who specializes in orthopedics	جَرّاح تَقويم العِظام
oscheal	relating to the scrotum (the pouch containing the testes and their accessory organs)	صَفَني
ossiculectomy	removal of one or more of the ossicles of the middle ear	استِئصال العُظيمة
osteitis	inflammation of bone	التِهاب العَظم
osteoarthritis	a chronic disease characterized by progressive degeneration of the cartilage of the joints	فِصالٌ عَظمي
osteocarcinoma	carcinoma with osseous metaplasia	سرَطانةٌ عَظميّة
osteoclasis	surgical fracture or refracture of a bone	نَقضُ العَظم
osteocyte	a branched cell embedded in the matrix of bone tissue	خَليّةٌ عَظميّة
osteogenic sarcoma	malignant bone sarcoma which arises from bone-forming cells and affects chiefly ends of long bones	ساركومةٌ عَظميّةٌ المَنشأ

Medical Words	Meaning in English	Meaning in Arabic
osteoma	a benign neoplasm of bone or bone tissue	وَرَمٌ عَظْمِيّ
osteomyelitis	inflammation of the bone marrow and adjacent bone	اِلْتِهاب العَظْم و النَّقْي
osteoporosis	reduction in the quantity of bone or atrophy of skeletal tissue	تَخَلْخُل العَظْم
otalgia	pain in the ear	أَلَمُ الأُذُن
otitis	inflammation of the ear	اِلْتِهاب الأُذُن
otorhinolaryngology	the branch of medicine dealing with the ear, nose, and throat	طِبُّ الأَنْف و الأُذُن و الحَنْجَرة
otoscopy	examination of the ear by means of an otoscope	تَنْظير الأُذُن
ovarian cyst	a benign or malignant growth on an ovary	كيسَة مَبيضِيَّة
ovariopathy	any disease of the ovary	اِعْتِلال مَبيضِيّ
ovariopexy	surgical fixation of the ovary to the abdominal wall	تَثْبيت المَبيض
ovoid	an oval or egg-shaped form	بَيضاوِيّ
ovulatory	relating to ovulation	إباضِيّ
oximeter	a device for measuring the oxygen saturation of arterial blood	مِقْياس التَأَكْسُج
palatine	relating to the palate: *the palatine tonsils*	حَنَكِيّ
palmar	relating to the palm of the hand	راحِيّ
palpebral	relating to the eyelid	جَفْنِيّ
pancreatic carcinoma	a malignant tumor in the pancreas	سَرَطان البِنكرياس
pancreatitis	inflammation of the pancreas	اِلْتِهاب البَنكرياس
panplegia	paralysis of all four extremities	شَلَل شامِل
parasympathomimetic	producing effects similar to those produced when a parasympathetic nerve is stimulated	مُحاكي اللاوُدِيّ
parathyroid gland	a small gland located at the posterior aspect of the thyroid gland, which regulates calcium	الغُدَد الدُرَيقِيَّة
parathyroidectomy	surgical removal of the parathyroid glands	اِسْتِئْصال الدُرَيقَة
parietal	pertaining to the walls of an organ or cavity	جِداريّ
parosmia	perversion of the sense of smell	خَطَل الشَمّ
patellectomy	excision of the patella (kneecap)	اِسْتِئْصال الرَضَفة
pathologist	a physician who practices, evaluates, or supervises diagnostic tests	اِخْتِصاصِيّ الباثولوجيا
pectoralgia	pain in the chest	أَلَم صَدْرِيّ
pediatrics	the medical specialty concerned with the study and treatment of children	طِبُّ الأَطْفال
pedograph	an instrument to record and study the gait (the manner or style of walking)	مُخَطِّط القَدَم
pelvic	pertaining to the hip bone	حَوْضِيّ
pelvimeter	an instrument for measuring the pelvis	مِقْياس الحَوْض
pelviscope	endoscopic instrument for examining the interior of the pelvis	تَنْظير الحَوْض
peribursal	surrounding a bursa (sacs of fluid near a joint)	مُحيط بالجِراب

Medical Words	Meaning in English	Meaning in Arabic
pericardium	fibroserous, double-layered membrane surrounding the heart	التامور
perineocele	a hernia in the perineum (the area between the opening of the vagina and the anus in a woman)	قَيلَةٌ عِجانِيّة
periosteum	a fibrous vascular membrane that covers bones	غِشاء العظم
peristalsis	the wave-like muscular contractions of the digestive tract	تَمَعُّج
peritoneal cavity	the potential space between the parietal and the visceral layers of the peritoneum	جَوفُ الصِّفاق
peritoneal dialysis	a method of reducing the levels of waste products in the blood in cases of kidney failure	ديالٌ صِفاقِيّ
peritonitis	an inflammation of the membrane which lines the inside of the abdomen and all of the internal organs	التِهاب الصِّفاق
phagocyte	any cell that ingests microorganisms or other cells and foreign particles	بُلعَمِيّة
phalangeal	relating to a phalanx (bones of fingers or toes)	سُلامِيّ
pharyngospasm	spasm of the muscles of the pharynx	تَشَنُّجُ البُلعُوم
pharyngotomy	incision of the pharynx	بَضعُ البُلعُوم
phlebitis	inflammation of a vein	التِهابٌ وَريدِيّ
phlebotomy	incision of a vein	فَصدٌ (بَضعُ الوَريد)
phonoscope	a device for recording heart sounds	مِجهارُ الحاكي
phonometer	an instrument for measuring the frequency and intensity of sounds	مِقياسُ الصَّوت
photangiophobia	an abnormal fear of photalgia (light)	رُهابُ الانبِهار
photophobia	abnormal sensitivity of the eyes to light	رُهابُ الضَّوء
phrenectomy	resection of a section of a phrenic nerve	استِئصالُ الحِجاب
phrenicotripsy	crushing of a section of the phrenic nerve	هَرسُ العَصَب الحِجابي
phrenitis	inflammation of the diaphragm	التِهاب الحِجاب
pilonidal	having a nidus of hairs	شَعرِيّ
plantar	pertaining to the sole of the foot	أخمَصِيّ
pleuritis	inflammation of the pleura (membrane surrounding the lungs)	التِهاب الجَنبَة
pleurocentesis	surgical puncture and drainage of the thoracic cavity	بَزلٌ جَنبِي (بَزلٌ صَدرِيّ)
pleurodesis	the production of adhesions between the visceral and pa-rietal pleurae	إلصاقٌ جَنبِي
pneumectomy	excision of lung tissue	استِئصالُ الرِّئة
pneumoconiosis	deposition of large amounts of dust or other particulate matter in the lungs	سُحار؛ تَغَبُّرُ الرِّئة
pneumonia	an infection of the lung	التِهابٌ رِئَوِيّ
podiatry	the branch of medicine that deals with the diagnosis, treatment, and prevention of diseases of the human foot	مَبحَثُ الأقدام
polydactyly	presence of more than five digits on hand or foot	عَدَش؛كَثرَةُ الأصابِع
polydipsia	excessive or abnormal thirst	عُطاش
polygraph	an instrument that simultaneously records changes in vari-ous physiological parameters (lie detector)	جِهازُ كَشف الكَذب

Medical Words	Meaning in English	Meaning in Arabic
polymorphous	occurring in more than one form	متعدد الأشكال
polyphagia	excessive eating	نَهام
polyspermia	excessive secretion of semen	غزارة المَني
posterior	directed toward or situated at the back	الخلفي
postmortem	occurring after death	تال للموت/ تشريح
postnatal	occurring after birth	تال للولادة
prenatal	preceding birth	سابق للولادة
primipara	a woman who has given birth for the first time	بكرية (حامل للمرة الأولى بجنين حي)
proctopexy	surgical fixation of a prolapsing rectum	تثبيت المَستقيم
prodrome	an early or premonitory symptom of a disease	بادرة
prognathic	pertaining to a forward relationship of the jaws	أفقَم
prognosis	prediction of the probable course and outcome of a disease	الإنذار،المآل
prolapse	the falling down or downward displacement of a part or viscus	تدلّي
prone position	a position in which the patient is lying face downward	وضعية الانكباب
prophylaxis	a measure taken to maintain health and prevent the spread of disease	اتقاء،توقية
prostatometer	instrument to measure the prostate	مقياس البروستاتة
prosthesis	an artificial substitute for a missing body part	بدلة
proximal	nearest to a point of reference	دان
pseudoplegia	false paralysis due to a conversion disorder	شلل كاذب
psychiatrist	a physician who specializes in mental disorders	طبيب نفسي
psychiatry	the branch of health science that deals with the study, treatment, and prevention of mental disorders	الطب النفسي
psychoactive	affecting the mind or behavior	نفسي المفعول/ النفساني
psychology	the science dealing with the mind and mental processes	علم النفس: السيكولوجيا
psychotropic	capable of affecting the mind, emotions, and behavior	نفسي التأثير
pubococcygeal	relating to the pubis and the coccyx	عاني عصعصي
pulmoaortic	relating to the pulmonary artery and the aorta	رئوي أبهري
pulmonary	pertaining to the lungs	رئوي
pyelogram	a radiograph or series of radiographs of the renal pelvis and ureter	صورة الحويضة
pyloroplasty	an elective surgical procedure of the lower portion of the stomach, the pylorus	رأب البواب
pyorrhea	purulent inflammation of the gums and tooth sockets	تقيح دواعم السن
pyuria	presence of pus in the urine	بيلة قيحية
quadriplegia	paralysis of all four limbs	شلل رباعي (شلل الأطراف الأربعة)
rachiocentesis	the act of piercing or penetrating with a pointed object	بزل سيسائي
radiculitis	inflammation of a spinal nerve root	التهاب الجذر
radiotherapy	treatment of disease with radiation	المعالجة الإشعاعية
rectocele	hernial protrusion of part of the rectum into the vagina	قيلة مستقيمية

Medical Words	Meaning in English	Meaning in Arabic
remission	abatement or lessening in severity of the symptoms of a disease	هدأة
renal	pertaining to the kidney	كلوي
reproductive	pertaining to the process of reproduction	توالدي إنجابي تناسلي
resection	surgical removal of all or part of an organ, tissue, or structure	قطع
respiratory	pertaining to respiration	تنفسي
reticulocyte	an immature red blood cell that contains a network of basophilic filaments	خلية شبكية
retinitis	inflammation of the retina	التهاب الشبكية
retinoschisis	splitting of the retina	انشقاق الشبكية
retrouterine	behind the uterus	خلف الرحم
retroversion	the tipping backward of an entire organ or part	انقلاب خلفي
rhabdoid	resembling a rod; rod shaped	عصوي
rhabdomyoma	a benign neoplasm derived from striated muscle	الورم العضلي المخطط
rhinitis	inflammation of the mucous lining of the nose	التهاب الأنف
rhinoplasty	plastic surgery of the nose	رأب الأنف
rhinoscopy	examination of the nose with a speculum	تنظير الأنف
right hypochondriac	pertaining to the right regions of the upper abdomen beneath the lower ribs and lateral to the epigastric region	مراقي الايمن
right iliac (inguinal)	pertaining to the right hip bone	الحرقفي الأيمن
right lateral recumbent	a position in which the patient lies on the right side with the upper knee and thigh drawn upward	رافد الجانبي الأيمن
right lower quadrant or RLQ	the region of the abdomen that contains the terminal ileum, appendix and cecum	الربع السفلي الأيمن
right lumbar	relating to the right loins, or the part of the back and sides between the ribs and the pelvis	القطني الأيمن
right upper quadrant or RUQ	the abdominal region that contains the liver, duodenum, and head of pancreas	الربع العلوي الأيمن
sacral (lower back)	relating to the sacrum	عجزي
sacrum	triangular bone at the base of the spine	عجزية
salpingectomy	surgical removal of the fallopian tube	استئصال البوق
salpingitis	inflammation of the fallopian tube	التهاب البوق (في الرحم)
salpingoscope	a device for examining the nasopharynx and the Eustachian tube	منظار النفير
schizophrenia	a heterogeneous psychiatric disorder	فصام
sclerectasia	a bulging state of the sclera (the tough, white outer coat of the eyeball)	اندلاق الصلبة
sclerosis	an induration or hardening	تصلب
scoliosis	abnormal lateral and rotational curvature of the vertebral column	جنف
scotometer	an instrument for diagnosing and measuring scotomas (an area of depressed vision in the visual field)	مقياس العتمة
seborrhea	excessive discharge from the sebaceous glands	مذت (مذت الرجل: ردي على جلده مثل الدهن)

Medical Words	Meaning in English	Meaning in Arabic
septicemia	systemic infection of the blood by pathogenic microorganisms	إنتان دَمَوي
septoplasty	a surgical procedure to correct the shape of the septum of the nose	رَأْبُ الحاجِزِ الأَنْفِيّ؛رَأْبُ الوَتيرة
septostomy	surgical creation of an opening in a septum (a wall or partition dividing a body space or cavity)	فَغْرُ الحاجِز
serology	the branch of science concerned with serum	السيرولوجيا؛عِلْمُ الأَمْصال
sialaadenitis	inflammation of a salivary gland	الْتِهابُ الغُدَّةِ اللُّعابِيَّة
sialogram	an X-ray image of the duct of a salivary gland	صورةُ القَناةِ اللُّعابِيَّة
sigmoidoscopy	direct examination of the interior of the sigmoid colon	تَنْظيرُ السِّينِيّ
Sims' (also known as left lateral) position	the patient on the left side and chest, the right knee and thigh drawn up, the left arm along the back	وَضْعِيَّةُ سيمز (وضعية اضطجاعية للفحص) المهبلي
sinusotomy	incision into a sinus	بَضْعُ الجَيب
somatesthesia	bodily sensation, the conscious awareness of the body	الحِسُّ المُشْتَرك
somatic	pertaining to or characteristic of the body	جَسَدِيّ
somatotropic	having a stimulating effect on body growth	مُوَجَّهٌ جَسَدِيّ
somnolence	drowsiness or sleepiness, particularly in excess	نُعَمُومَة
sphygmomanometer	an instrument for measuring arterial blood pressure	مِقْياسُ ضَغْطِ الدَّم (الشِّرياني)
spinal	pertaining to a spine	شَوْكِيّ (مُتَعَلِّق ببنية تشريحية مؤتلفة)
spinal (vertebral) cavity	the cavity that contains the spinal cord	تجويف الشوكي
spirometer	an instrument for measuring air inhaled into and exhaled out of the lungs	مِقْياسُ التَّنَفُّس
splenectomy	the surgical removal of the spleen (a large, highly vascular lymphoid organ)	اسْتِئْصالُ الطِّحال
splenomegaly	enlargement of the spleen	تَضَخُّمُ الطِّحال؛طِحَل
splenoptosis	downward displacement of the spleen	تَدَلِّي الطِّحال
splenorrhagia	hemorrhage from a ruptured spleen	نَزْفُ الطِّحال
spondylitis	inflammation of one or more vertebrae	الْتِهابُ الفَقار
spondylosis	ankylosis of a vertebral joint	تَنَكُّسُ الفَقار
steatorrhea	an excessive amount of fat in the stool	إسْهالٌ دُهْنِيّ
stenosis	an abnormal narrowing or contraction of a body passage	تَضَيُّق
sternad	toward the sternum	باتِّجاه القَصّ
stethoscope	any of various instruments used for listening to sounds produced within the body	سمّاعَة
subchondriac	pertaining to under the cartilage of the ribs	تحت الغضروف
subchoroidal	below the choroid coat of the eye	تَحْتَ المَشيميَّة (في العين وفي البطينات) الدماغية
subcostal	below a rib	تَحْتَ الضِّلْع
subcutaneous	beneath the skin	تَحْتَ الجِلْد
sublingual	below the tongue	تَحْتَ اللِّسان
sudoresis	profuse sweating	تَعَرُّقٌ غَزير
suicidal	pertaining to suicide or prone to suicide	انْتِحار
superficial (external)	situated on or near the surface	سَطْحِيّ

Medical Words	Meaning in English	Meaning in Arabic
superior (cranial)	situated nearer the vertex of the head	عُلْوِيّة
supine position	lying on the back	وَضْعِيّة الاسْتِلْقاء
supracerebellar	on or above the surface of the cerebellum	فَوْق المُخَيْخ
suprapelvic	above the pelvis	فَوْق الحَوْض
supraventricular	situated or occurring above the ventricles	فَوْق البُطَيْن
sympathomimetic	denoting mimicking of action of the sympathetic system	مُحاكي الوَدّيّ
tachycardia	abnormally rapid heart rate	تَسَرُّع القَلْب
tendinitis	the inflammation of a tendon, a tough rope-like tissue that connects muscle to bone	التِهاب الوَتَر
tenodesis	suture of the end of a tendon to a bone	خِياطَة الوَتَر (بالعَظْم)
testosterone	male hormone produced by the testes and (in small amounts) in the ovaries	تِستوستيرون [هرمون]
thalamotomy	a surgical procedure that destroys part of a large oval area of gray matter within the brain	بَضْع المِهاد
thermometer	an instrument for measuring temperature	مِقْياس الحَرارة
thoracentesis	surgical puncture and drainage of the thoracic cavity	بَزْل الصَّدْر
thoracic (chest)	pertaining to the chest	صَدْرِيّ
thoracic cavity	the space within the thoracic walls	جَوْف الصَّدْر
thoracoschisis	congenital fissure of the thoracic wall	انْشِقاق الصَّدْر
thoracotomy	incision of the chest wall	بَضْع الصَّدْر
thrombocyte	clotting cells	صَفيحَة
thrombocytosis	a blood disorder in which the body produces a surplus of platelets	كَثْرَة الصُّفَيْحات
thrombolytic	dissolving or splitting up a thrombus	حالّ الخَثْرة
thrombosis	formation or presence of a thrombus (blood clot)	خَثار
thymectomy	removal of the thymus gland	اسْتِئْصال التُّوثة
thymopathy	any disease of the thymus (a ductless gland lying in the upper mediastinum)	اعْتِلال التُّوثة
thyroadenitis	inflammation of the thyroid	التِهاب الغُدّة الدَّرَقِيّة
thyrotoxic	pertaining to the effects of thyroid hormone excess	مُتعلِق بالتَّسَمُّم الدَّرَقيّ
tibiofemoral	pertaining to the tibia (the inner and larger of the two bones of the lower leg) and femur (thigh bone)	ظُنْبوبيّ فَخْذيّ
tonsillar	pertaining to a tonsil	لَوْزيّ
tonsillectomy	surgical removal of tonsils	اسْتِئْصال اللَّوْزَتين
tracheostomy	surgical construction of an opening in the trachea	فَغْر الرُّغامَى
tracheotome	an instrument for incising the trachea	مِبْضَع الرُّغامَى
tracheotomy	incision of the trachea	بَضْع الرُّغامَى
transdermal	across the skin	بطَريق الأَدَمة/ عبر الجلد
transfusion	the process of transferring whole blood or blood components from one person (donor) to another	نَقْل الدَّم
transurethral	performed through the urethra (the membranous canal through which urine is discharged from the bladder to the exterior of the body)	بطَريق الإحْليل

Medical Words	Meaning in English	Meaning in Arabic
trichophagia	the compulsive eating of hair	أكْل الشَّعْر
trigonitis	inflammation of the trigone region of the bladder	الْتِهاب الْمُثَلَّث الْمَثانيّ
tympanic	pertaining or belonging to a tympanum (eardrum)	طبلي
tympanoplasty	surgical repair or reconstruction of the middle ear	رأب الطَّبْلَة
ulnocarpal	relating to the ulna and the carpus, or to the ulnar side of the wrist	زَنديّ رُسْغيّ
umbilical	resembling a navel or an umbilical cord	سُرّيّ
ungual	pertaining to the nails	ظُفْريّ
unilateral	pertaining to one side	وَحيد الْجانِب
uremia	the presence of excessive amounts of urea and other waste products in the blood	تبوّل الدَّم
ureterectasis	distention of the ureter (the tube that leads from the kidney to the urinary bladder)	تَوَسُّع الْحالِب
urethrostenosis	constriction of the urethra (a tube that leads from the urinary bladder to the outside of the body)	تَضَيُّق الإحْليل
urinary system	the bodily system consisting of the organs that produce, collect, and eliminate urine and including the kidneys, ureters, urinary bladder, and urethra	الْجِهاز الْبَوْليّ
urodynia	pain accompanying urination	وَجَع التَّبَوُّل
urologist	a physician specialized in diagnosing and treating diseases of the genitourinary tract	جَرّاح الْجِهاز الْبَوْليّ
uroscopy	examination of the urine, usually by means of a microscope	فَحْص الْبَوْل
uterine	relating to the uterus (the hollow muscular organ in female mammals)	تَطْبيل الرَّحِم
uteroplasty	plastic surgery of the uterus	رأب الرَّحِم
uveitis	inflammation of the uveal tract: iris, ciliary body, and choroid	الْتِهاب الْعِنَبِيَّة
uvulotome	an instrument for cutting the uvula (any hanging, fleshy mass)	مِبْضَع اللَّهاة
vaginitis	inflammation of the vagina	الْتِهاب الْمَهْبِل
valvar	relating to a valve	صِمامي
valvuloplasty	plastic surgery to repair a valve, especially a heart valve	رأب الصِّمام
varicocele	an abnormal enlargement of the veins which drain the testicles	قَيْلَة دَواليَّة
vascular	relating to or containing blood vessels	وِعائي
vasculitis	inflammation of a blood vessel	الْتِهاب وِعائي
vasodepressor	having the effect of lowering the blood pressure through reduction in peripheral resistance	خافِض للتَّوَتُّر الوِعائي
vasodilation	widening of the lumen of blood vessels	تَوَسُّع الأوْعِيَة
vasostomy	surgical formation of an opening into the ductus (vas) deferens (the secretory duct of the testis)	فَغْر الأسْهَر
venous	relating to a vein	وَريدي
ventral (anterior)	pertaining to the abdomen or to any venter	بَطْني/أمامي
ventral cavity	the body cavity composed of the thoracic, abdominal, and pelvic cavities	جوف الْبَطْن

Medical Words	Meaning in English	Meaning in Arabic
venulitis	inflammation of the venules	التهاب الوريدي
vertebral	pertaining to a vertebra	فَقَري
vesical	pertaining to or emanating from the urinary bladder	مَثاني
vesiculogram	a radiograph of the seminal vesicles	صورة الحُوَيصِلة
vestibulotomy	operation for an opening into the vestibule of the labyrinth (the internal ear)	بَضع الدَهليز (الأذني)
visceral	relating to the viscera (the soft internal organs of the body)	حَشَوي
vulvitis	inflammation of the vulva (the external genitals of the female)	التهاب الفَرج
xenograft	a graft transferred from an animal of one species to one of another species	طُعم أجنبي (طُعم غيرَوي)
xeroderma	excessive dryness of the skin	جَفاف الجِلد
xerosis	dryness of the skin	جَفاف
xerostomia	a dryness of the mouth	جَفاف الفَم
xiphoid (process)	the cartilage at the lower end of the sternum	سَيفي الشَّكُل الناتئ الرُهابي (الرُهابة)

Index